boosting
immunity

boosting
immunity

creating wellness naturally

len saputo, m.d.
nancy faass, m.s.w., m.p.h.
editors

new world library
novato, california

New World Library
14 Pamaron Way
Novato, California 94949

Copyright © 2002 by Len Saputo, M.D., and Nancy Faass, M.S.W., M.P.H.
Editorial by Katharine Farnam Conolly
Front cover design by Mary Beth Salmon
Text design and typography by Tona Pearce Myers

The material in this book is intended for educational purposes. It is not meant to take the place of diagnosis and treatment by a qualified medical practitioner or therapist. No expressed or implied guarantee as to the effects of the use of the recommendations can be given nor liability taken.

Grateful acknowledgment is given to the following publishers for permission to reprint portions of the following materials in *Boosting Immunity:* Chapters 5, 9, and 11 of the present work are adapted from chapters 20, 23, and 43 of *Optimal Digestion* by Trent W. Nichols, M.D. and Nancy Faass, M.S.W., M.P.H., copyright © 1999 by Nancy Faass, M.S.W., M.P.H. Reprinted by permission of HarperCollins Publishers, Inc.; Chapters 6 and 10 of the present work are adapted from chapter 9 of *The Food Allergy Cure* by Dr. Ellen W. Cutler. Copyright © 2001 by Dr. Ellen W. Cutler. Reprinted by permission of Harmony Books, a division of Random House, Inc.

Library of Congress Cataloging-in-Publication Data
Saputo, Len, and Nancy Faass.
Boosting immunity : balancing your body's ecology for maximum health /
by Len Saputo and Nancy Faass.
    p.   cm.
Includes bibliographical references and index.
ISBN 1-57731-127-2
1. Natural immunity. 2. Health. I. Title.
QR185.2 .S27 2002
616.07'9—dc21   2001005891

First Printing, February 2002
ISBN 1-57731-127-2
Printed in Canada on acid-free, recycled paper
Distributed to the trade by Publishers Group West

10 9 8 7 6 5 4 3

To the medical profession and all those connected with it, who dedicate their lives to health and healing.

contents

CHAPTER ONE

Creating Strong Immunity through Lifestyle

Len Saputo, M.D., and
Nancy Faass, M.S.W., M.P.H.

Everything you do — everything you touch, breathe, eat, and think affects your immunity. Everything! How you live your life is the most powerful resource known for preserving and restoring your immunity. Factors such as sleep, exercise, nutrition, stress reduction, and spiritual connection provide the foundation for a strong immune response. This information can be translated into practical steps you can take to enjoy a life of greater health and vitality.

A healthy lifestyle is also a *natural* way to build your immunity. This involves approaches that are simple, inexpensive, and safe — and that really work. You can become highly skilled at fine-tuning your lifestyle to produce maximum health. And these changes can be incorporated into your daily life gradually, at your own pace.

The beneficial effects of lifestyle on immunity have been documented in thousands of research studies. These studies come from a wide range of disciplines, from universities and medical centers around the world. This research has rediscovered the importance of the "style" in which we live our lives, and highlights its potential to enhance our overall health. In the following chapters we will explore some of this research and offer practical suggestions on how to apply it in your own life.

The Wellness Factor

The strength of the immune system is always a factor whenever there is illness — whether it's the common cold or cancer. It's the missing part of the equation we tend to overlook. You have probably experienced cycles in your life when you seemed to catch everything that came along. At other times, you may have remained perfectly healthy while those around you became ill. Your ability to resist illness is a yardstick that measures the strength of your immune system. The strength of your immunity can have a profound impact on whether you get sick, how long you stay sick, and how ill you become. So the immune reserves you build through a healthy lifestyle provide a buffer that will help to prevent or minimize illness.

Building Good Resistance

New information suggests that infections can leave us vulnerable to more serious conditions if they deplete our immunity.[1] This is important, because it can no longer be assumed that colds, flu, and other common illnesses are always harmless. Cryptosporidium is a case in point. In response to a recent outbreak in Canada, health officials said that most people who suffered from this flu-like illness would probably recover within two weeks.[2] However, they warned that the same microbe could be more harmful to people who had weakened immune function. Generally, those most vulnerable are young children, older people, and those with chronic health conditions. Understanding immunity and susceptibility can aid us in maintaining good health and strong resistance.

The Centers for Disease Control has repeatedly advised of the rising incidence of infectious diseases. A recent news article on a meningitis outbreak in the San Francisco Bay Area reflects how vulnerable we may become when immune function is compromised. When a form of meningitis was contracted by a number of children in northern California this year, a local public health officer pointed out the risk involved: "This is not an outbreak. Fifty to 60 percent of the population carries [strep] bacteria in their throats. Normally, it's not a problem, but if someone had a prior cold, and their body can't combat it, then it [could become] serious."[3]

These infections were not caused by exotic supergerms. They were the result of the overgrowth of potentially dangerous bacteria that normally coexist within us. Staph bacteria are another example of microbes that most of us carry. Like strep, these resident bacteria aren't usually a problem, because a healthy immune system will keep their growth in check. This is one of the reasons why severe illness from strep and staph is relatively rare. However, under certain circumstances, they can cause dangerous secondary infections, so they are to be taken seriously. Meningitis (which can result from strep infection) causes long-term damage in one out of four cases. The threat of these types of bacterial infections clearly demonstrates why it is so important to build robust immunity.

New Research

For the past fifteen years, extensive research has deepened our understanding of immunity, particularly through the enormous number of studies on cancer and AIDS. Science has made great strides in the exploration of how the immune system works and how to enhance its function. As a result, the American public has a greater appreciation for the importance of immunity.

There is also a large body of medical literature that documents the role of lifestyle factors in immunity. This research reflects the impact on our health of the things we do every day. It also provides information we can use to modify our lifestyle, in order to enhance health and immune function. We will explore some of this research and offer practical suggestions for applying it.

Lifestyle and Immunity

To explore the effects of lifestyle on immunity, consider the example of the common cold. Our vulnerability depends on the balance between the strength of our immunity and the strength of the threatening virus.[4] Once exposed, we only get sick if our immune defenses are inadequate. When our reserve defenses are depleted, they can no longer prevent the virus from invading our cells. We all know that when our defenses are strong, we almost never get sick.

Yet many of us tend to overestimate our ability to resist illness, and in the process we neglect our health. Most of us don't get enough rest. We often eat on the run. We may be exposed to a variety of germs and toxins daily. And, for most of us, stress has become a way of life. We frequently take better care of our cars than of our bodies. It doesn't take a research scientist to figure out why we sometimes get sick.

Consider the effects of lifestyle on our susceptibility to illness. The factors that may increase our vulnerability to disease can also be modified to improve our resistance.

- *Rest and rejuvenation.* How often have you caught a cold after not getting enough sleep? We depend on adequate restful sleep to restore our bodies and refresh our minds. During deep sleep, our bodies release potent immune-enhancing substances that strengthen immune function. It is especially important to get additional rest when we are ill.
- *Exercise.* We need regular exercise. The body has a remarkable ability to increase its metabolic capacity through consistent regular physical conditioning. We all know how invigorated and strong we feel when we're in shape. Overall fitness creates reserve capacity that not

only serves as a buffer against disease but also helps us recover more quickly.

- *Good nutrition.* A healthy diet is absolutely essential to maintain good immunity. Food provides our cells with the raw materials they require to meet the body's needs. We tend to take nutrition for granted, believing that we'll get along just fine, even if we don't consume all the nutrition we need. Yet we shouldn't assume that just because we live in a modern society we have adequate nutrition. Hundreds of in-depth studies have documented that malnutrition exists in industrialized nations today, among both the rich and poor.

  Widespread nutritional factors that can compromise our immune capacity include eating too much sugar or starch, obesity, high cholesterol, and the regular use of alcohol. If the immune system is malnourished, it may not have the resources needed to protect us against illness. A healthy immune system depends on adequate amounts of vitamins, minerals, and other important metabolic nutrients. For example, the vast majority of our immune function is dependent on vitamin A and zinc, nutrients that are often lacking in the modern diet.

- *Toxins and pollution.* The metabolic machinery of our cells is exquisitely sensitive to many toxins that can interfere with the body's normal biochemical processes. Every day we are exposed to thousands (yes, thousands) of chemicals in our food, water, and air that were nonexistent until the Industrial Revolution of the nineteenth and twentieth centuries. As a result, our bodies must cope with manufactured chemicals, pesticides, heavy metals, petroleum products, and plastics that can accumulate in our tissues and that are toxic to the immune system. Clearing the body of these environmental toxins increases our requirement for antioxidants and various other nutrients. Because of these exposures, our nutritional requirements may be increased to higher levels than we can obtain in our diet, making it important to use nutritional supplements to remain healthy. And because of the prevalence of these exposures, it's also important to build detoxification into our lifestyle.

Some toxic chemicals have been documented to cause coldlike symptoms. A committee of the World Health Organization reported that up to 30 percent of new and remodeled buildings emit air pollutants such as formaldehyde, asbestos, volatile chemicals, and other toxins and allergens. The effects of these emissions can cause "sick building syndrome."[5] Solutions to the chemical sensitivity that may result include avoiding the sources of exposure, detoxifying the body and, when necessary, getting treatment from a physician trained in environmental medicine.

- *The stress factor.* There is now strong data that documents the impact of stress on immunity and susceptibility to illness.[6] For instance, remember how many of your friends caught colds during final exams? A report of 276 volunteers exposed to a common cold virus showed that those who had been under stress for more than a month were most likely to get sick.[7] In another study, children with a history of stress and recurrent colds were found to have lower localized immunity.[8] Stress has also been found to stimulate immune-suppressing chemicals such as adrenaline.[9] Fortunately, research has found that stress reducers such as meditation, relaxation, guided imagery, and hypnosis can effectively enhance immunity.[10]

What's in This Book

All these interactions with our environment — including water, air, food, toxins, and stress — have an enormous influence on our ability to stay healthy. In the chapters that follow, we will consider the impact of each of these factors on our body and how they can impair or enhance immune function. Practical solutions for building immunity will be suggested by a team of experts in internal medicine, nutrition, environmental medicine, and alternative and complementary therapies, including:

- Getting the ideal amount of sleep
- The beneficial effects of water
- The impact of nutrition and digestion on immunity
- Clearing the body of allergens and toxins to enhance health
- The mind-body-spirit connection to immunity and well-being

This basic information can be applied in day-to-day living. When you are under stress, you can use these resources to restore balance. This will provide you with a great sense of control over your own health. These tools are intended for anyone interested in prevention and also for the millions of Americans who suffer from chronic illness.

We are all in awe of the great technological advances in medicine over the past fifty years. In the midst of this technological era, science is also rediscovering that lifestyle is a fundamental determinant of good health. Drawing on the best of research and medical practice, each chapter in the book will provide practical strategies you can use to achieve vibrant health.

- *Preventing illness.* You'll find information that will help you stay well and get well faster if you're sick.
- *Improving a chronic condition.* All these strategies are potentially valuable for restoring health. Immunity is always a piece of the puzzle whenever there is illness.

- *Finding a healthy diet.* We offer an approach that is simple, sensible, and backed by an enormous amount of research. This will take some of the guesswork out of what to eat and why.
- *Gaining new tools for health.* The book draws from a variety of disciplines in medicine and natural health, providing you with a range of options.
- *An individualized approach.* Suggestions will be included throughout on how to personalize these strategies to meet your unique needs.

We are entering an era in which the focus of health care is shifting to self-care. The importance of lifestyle is becoming increasingly apparent. We hope that you will select the approaches that best fit your needs. Our goal here is to provide solutions for the whole person — body, mind, and spirit. Practical strategies will be suggested for strengthening your resistance to illness and enhancing your health.

Be well.

$\mathcal{S}$

Len Saputo, M.D., is founder and director of the Health Medicine Forum, and non-profit educational foundation. Over the past seven years, he has guided the development of an integrative, holistic model of health care, which is person-centered and focused on prevention. He is also the medical director of the Health Medicine Institute (HMI) located in Walnut Creek, California, an integrative medicine center that is bringing this model into clinical practice. Further information on this approach and on the Forum are available on the Web at www.healthmedicine.org. Consultations with Dr. Saputo can be arranged by calling HMI at (925) 937-9550.

Dr. Saputo is active in public education on holistic health through radio, television, the Forum's monthly presentations, and his own speaking engagements. Information on his appearances and radio program can be obtained on the Forum's website listed above. He is also an avid tennis player and is currently ranked number on in the world in senior men's singles by the International Tennis Federation.

~

Nancy Faass, M.S.W., M.P.H., is a writer and editor in San Francisco who provides book and project development in integrative medicine and the social sciences. With a master's degree in public health from the University of California at Berkeley and a master's in social work from Catholic University in Washington, D.C., she has worked as a science editor at the University of California, San Francisco (U.C.S.F.), as an archivist, and in scholarly publishing. She has served as a program coordinator in both social services and in education. Ms. Faass is developer and editor of *Integrating Complementary Medicine into Health Systems.* She is also codeveloper and coeditor of *Optimal Digestion* from HarperCollins with Trent Nichols, M.D.

Notes

1. C. Burress et al., "Two More Cases of Meningitis in Bay Area. Berkeley Girl a Possible Link," *San Francisco Chronicle,* Chronicle Sections, 12 May, 2001.

2. F. J. Frost et al., "Serological Analysis of a Cryptosporidiosis Epidemic," *International Journal of Epidemiology* 29, no. 2 (April 2000): 376–79.

3. Please see note 1 above.

4. M. J. Makela et al., "Viruses and Bacteria in the Etiology of the Common Cold," *Journal of Clinical Microbiology* 36, no. 2 (February 1998) 539–43.

5. J. Thraser and A. Broughton, *The Poisoning of Our Homes and Workplaces* (Santa Ana, Calif.: Seadora, Inc., 1989).

6. J. K. Kiecolt-Glaser and R. Glaser, "Psychoneuroimmunology: Can Psychological Interventions Modulate Immunity?" *Journal of Consulting Clinical Psychology* 60 (1992): 569–75.

7. S. Cohen et al., "Types of Stressors That Increase Susceptibility to the

Common Cold in Healthy Adults," *Health Psychology* 17, no. 3 (May 1998): 214–33.

8. P. D. Drummond and B. Hewson-Bower, "Increased Psychosocial Stress and Decreased Mucosal Immunity in Children with Recurrent Upper Respiratory Tract Infections," *Journal of Psychosomatic Research* 43, no. 3 (September 1997): 271–78.

9. M. Irwin et al., "Reduction of Immune Function in Life Stress and Depression," *Biological Psychology* 27 (1990): 22–30.

10. M. Rossman, M.D., *Guided Imagery for Self-Healing* (Novato, Calif.: Kramer/New World Library, 2000).

the
basics

CHAPTER TWO

Immunity Made Easy

Michael Rosenbaum, M.D.

Megan was the perfect kindergarten teacher, but she seemed to be sick all the time. In the beginning, she loved her work and was usually up early and out of the house by 6:30. She often devoted part of each evening to lesson planning or preparing projects for the children. Over time she noticed that she was becoming more and more susceptible to colds and infections. Her doctor indicated that she was probably working too hard and being exposed to a broad array of germs in the classroom. Still, she was able to keep up until the layoffs began at her school. The program was totally reorganized, and although her job survived the cuts, the tension at work placed her under severe stress. That winter, she noticed that her resistance was lower, and she seemed to catch everything that was going around. The infections became more frequent and lasted longer.

The holidays were the last straw. She got the flu, followed by strep throat, and then a stomach virus. Feeling tired and listless, she began having frequent low-grade fevers. She wondered if she would ever get her energy back. Her fatigue made it almost impossible to exercise, and some days it was difficult to function at work. It was also hard to concentrate. Somehow she avoided going out on disability leave — she was able to carry on, although it seemed as though she dragged through each day.

She would go home at 4:00 each day and collapse. It took the whole weekend to recuperate and store up enough energy for the week ahead. Megan knew she needed to break the cycle. She sought the help of an allergist who practiced integrative medicine, using nutrition and lifestyle interventions in combination with medication and traditional allergy treatment.

The doctor suggested she minimize her exposure to germs by washing her hands frequently. She had been unaware of how often she had been picking up bacterial and viral infections just from hugging the children and then touching her eyes or nose. He also encouraged her to simplify her life and reduce the stress as much as possible.

Certain foods and supplements were recommended to strengthen her immune system. He pointed out that sleep is very important and that people who don't sleep sometimes find that their immunity is suppressed. Specific nutrients and herbs were prescribed to stimulate her immune function and within a few weeks she found that she was quite well again.

Immune Defenses

Our immunity is a system of vast defenses fighting a never-ending war to protect us against invading microbes in our food, water, and the air we breath. These defensive efforts are extensive and sophisticated. Imagine a system with a trillion components — a million armies, each with a million troops.

These defenses are present in all life and surprisingly similar in most mammals. Two basic types of immunity have evolved: general immunity, which provides immediate defenses against any invader, and specific immunity, which is targeted against particular infections we've encountered in the past.

General immunity. The innate immunity we're born with reacts to anything in the body perceived as foreign or threatening, whether it's a microbe or an allergenic food. As part of this protection, various types of cells are strategically located throughout the body that respond in our defense immediately, regardless of the attacker or the circumstance.

Specific immunity. Some of our immune defenses are programmed to pursue and attack only microbes or food that they recognize. Every time we're exposed to a particular illness or receive a vaccination, our immune system remembers that exposure. If any of these bacteria or viruses attempt to bother us again, the immune systems calls up cells that function as troops or artillery, targeted specifically at that offender. So if you had the flu last year, your immune memory would recognize that particular virus and muster up various defenses to protect you. If the strain of flu you're exposed to is different than the one you previously had, your system will be unable to recognize it or respond. That's when general immunity is so important. (See the following table for specifics on the major players in your immune system.)

The Players in Your Immune System

The Assault Force

THE OLD GUARD

Phagocytes	Roam the blood stream and other body fluids; can engulf and consume microbes
Macrophages and Neutrophils	Two types of phagocytes; some can identify invaders who have history of causing harm

T CELLS: THE DEMOLITION SQUAD

T helpers	Amplify the immune response
T suppressors	Calm the immune system, once the threat of infection is over
Natural killer cells	Roam the bloodstream and the fluids of the body to protect us; attack viruses or tumors by injecting them with poisonous toxins
Killer cells (Cytotoxic T cells)	Also destroy tumors or cells that contain specific viruses

Antibody Artillery

B CELLS AND ANTIBODIES

B cells	Mature into plasma cells, which make antibodies
Plasma cells	Make antibodies: IgA, SIgA, IgE, IgG, IgM
Antibodies	Protein arrows that help trap microbes and allergenic food particles

In sum, three of the primary components of the immune system are:

- *Scavenger cells.* General defenses that police the body and devour microbes
- *T cells.* Some command the immune response; others poison microbes
- *Antibodies.* Microscopic arrows made of protein, targeted at microbes or allergenic foods.

The Assault Forces

The Old Guard

Our generalized immune defenses include a protective system that is found in the immunity of most all animal life and has evolved over millions of years. These scavenger cells have a long history as the guardians and defenders of our immune system.

- *Phagocytes* are the loyal foot soldiers of the immune system. They roam the body and defend us against any type of invader — whether it's bacteria, viruses, mold, debris of dead cells, or undigested food.
- *Macrophages* are a type of phagocyte that ingest, swallow, and destroy potentially harmful microbes. Some are highly specialized cells whose sole purpose is to process and label new invaders. When they identify a "dangerous" microbe, they then alert the T cells. This surveillance activity of the macrophages initiates the entire immune response.

The macrophage, viewed through an electron microscope, resembles a big blue shag rug. Photographed in the process of swallowing a yeast cell, the macrophage looks more like the Cookie Monster on Sesame Street than a member of an elite defensive force.

T Cells: The Demolition Squad

T cells are another member of the assault force of the immune system. The "T" in T cells refers to the thymus, a gland in the chest just behind the breastbone where the T cells "grow up" and are "trained" for their future role in our protection.

- *Natural killer cells.* These T cells function like a demolition force. When they identify a tumor or virus, they punch a hole in its cell wall and pump in toxins manufactured from oxygen — peroxide, nitric acid, or hypochlorite (very similar to laundry bleach).
- *Cytotoxic T cells.* Also known as "killer cells," they use a similar method of demolition, but since they have specific memory, they're targeted against particular viruses or against tumors.

T Cells: Command Central

Other important types of T cells are those that act as commanders, giving the order to fight or call off the battle.

- *T helper cells* activate or "upregulate" the entire immune response. There are millions of T helpers in the body. Each one carries the memory of a past encounter with an infection-causing microbe — defined as a pathogen. If the T helper cell bumps into a pathogenic microbe, the T cell promptly clones itself into an army of cells and signals a call to arms.

T helpers even carry blueprints for the plan of attack.

- Some T helpers call up armies of cells such as the killer cells — described as *cellular immunity.*
- Other T helpers signal attack by the immune artillery — the antibodies — also known as *humoral immunity.*

In cases of AIDS, the HIV virus destroys the T helper cells, eliminating the commanders of the immune army and shutting off the alarm system at the same time.

- *T suppressors* calm or "downregulate" immunity once the threat of infection is over. Like good governance, this provides a natural system of checks and balances in the body's immune defenses.

At thirty-five, Janice was one of the youngest executives in her field. She earned this distinction by working twelve hours or more a day and had done so ever since college. On one of her marathon business trips, she picked up a flu that she couldn't shake. Weeks later, she was still feeling exhausted, with a low-grade fever, a sore throat, and swollen glands. After six months, her energy hadn't returned and the doctor encouraged her to see a psychologist for stress management.

She continually battled exhaustion, sore muscles and joints, and bouts of pain. At times it was difficult to think clearly, and her memory seemed to be slipping. She began to develop allergies and became highly sensitive to a number of foods. Her digestion deteriorated. Little by little, she was losing her ability to function and eventually cut back on her work hours. Soon it became clear that she could no longer work.

When she sought a second opinion, her new doctor, an integrative physician, suggested that she may have chronic fatigue syndrome. He explained that this is a term that describes symptoms that can be caused by any number of conditions, including several caused by viruses — Epstein-Barr (mononucleosis), CMV (cytomegalovirus), and herpes 6. Although she was hopeful that she could return to work, he cautioned that up to 50 percent of patients with these conditions become disabled and permanently unable to work. In addition, fibromyalgia with its accompanying muscle aches and pains, is associated in nine out of ten cases.

Janice made major accommodations in her lifestyle to minimize stress and overexertion. She carefully organized her day and put together a support system that enabled her to accomplish the essentials. The doctor ordered blood tests to evaluate her immune function, which indicated that her T cell levels were lower than normal — particularly the T helper cells. The tests results also showed a profile suggestive of an active infection. Like many cases of chronic fatigue, the lab work did not provide a specific diagnosis, although her symptoms resembled those of a viral infection.

At this point, Janice found that even walking around the block was exhausting and stressful. Her doctor encouraged her to moderate her activity. He also prescribed nutrients and herbs to support her immune response in a program designed very specifically to meet her needs. He cautioned her that their initial goal should simply be to stabilize her condition and prevent her from getting worse. Once her health stopped declining, they were able to work toward gradual improvement. Although she wasn't able to resume her fast-paced lifestyle, she was able to achieve better quality of life.

Immune Defenses

Immune Artillery: Antibodies

Our protective immunity includes a specialized type of artillery — antibodies. These are microscopic protein arrows that can bombard germs such as bacteria and viruses. The bacteria they target are typically hundreds of times larger than the antibodies that pepper its surface, coating it with a sticky covering that resembles Velcro. This can trap and immobilize the bacteria in the body's mucus. For example, bacteria that we inhale may be caught in nasal mucus and discarded in a sneeze. Bacteria in our food may be entrapped in the mucus that lines the digestive tract, which functions like a slow conveyer belt, gradually carrying food and bacteria through the digestive process.

Antibodies also protect us from food allergens. When large undigested food molecules or allergenic foods are encountered, they are "glued" together by the antibodies to form a clump, described as an "immune complex." Like the bad bugs, the potentially harmful food is trapped, immobilized, and discarded.

The antibodies are classified by the letters of the alphabet, so our first line of defense is identified as antibody A. Antibodies are described as immune globulins (abbreviated as Ig), so immunoglobulin A is written as IgA. If you have allergies, you're likely to hear your doctor talk about IgE — the antibodies that trigger intense allergic reactions and can even be life threatening. IgG is associated with the antibodies that cause delayed reactions that are often described as sensitivities rather than true allergies.

Antibodies as Peacekeepers

These microscopic artillery also serve as the major peacekeeping force of the immune system. This is no small task. When we eat, an enormous amount of bacteria is unknowingly ingested in our food. Tremendous vigilance is involved in keeping these invaders under control, since we consume several pounds of food over the course of a day and tons of food a year. So we need huge quantities of antibodies to respond to these threats.

But the job doesn't end there. In addition, there are literally trillions of resident bacteria that make up our natural microflora in the digestive tract. The flora play a role in digestion and even manufacture certain essential nutrients. The antibodies must keep that ecology in balance and prevent any one type of bacteria or yeast (such as candida) from taking over in an "overgrowth" condition.

So the antibodies in the digestive tract have a daunting mission — they must identify the beneficial flora and leave them unharmed, while immobilizing the harmful bacteria — in a population of trillions. And all this effort must be accomplished peacefully, without causing inflammation, swelling, or soreness. Otherwise, we'd be doubled over in pain every time our immune system identified a little bacteria in our food. This highly sophisticated immune function is now considered the largest focus of immunity in the body, even greater than our T cells and other defenses.

Immune Artillery — The Antibodies

Type and location	Task	Effect
SIgA — in the lungs and digestive and urinary tracts	Targets any invader	Adheres to and immobilizes microbes and allergenic foods
IgA — in the bloodstream	Attacks specific microbes	An immune protector whose role is less understood
IgE — in the bloodstream and certain organs	Reacts to specific allergenic foods and substances	Causes sneezing and runny nose — defensive efforts to remove the allergen
IgG — in the bloodstream	Targeted against microbes that have made us ill in the past	Major infection-fighting antibody in the bloodstream
IgM — in the bloodstream and body secretions	Targets new infections, the first time encountered	Initial response within three to five days of exposure

Jim had always had a responsible job, good health, and lots of energy. At seventy-two, he had rarely been ill. Then his wife died and the nonprofit where he volunteered shut their doors. This triggered a major bout of depression, which had a suppressing effect on his immune system. He began to succumb to frequent infections. He developed his first case of pneumonia ever and was admitted to the hospital.

Jim had heard that older people tend to have reduced immunity. His doctor had mentioned that since most people eat less as they age and often don't completely absorb what they eat, they begin developing nutritional deficiencies. This creates a kind of chain reaction. As the body's stores of vitamin A and zinc become depleted, the immune system becomes less functional.

Dehydration can also become a problem. Whenever Jim threw up or had diarrhea, he tended to get dehydrated. Since he was sick, he couldn't replenish nutrients because he wasn't eating as well. This created a vicious cycle. Jim was getting worse and worse and because he was not longer active, he became more depressed.

Jim's doctor focused initially on combating the infection. Once it was under control, Jim's immune function was evaluated through blood tests. Then the doctor prescribed specific nutrients to support and rebuild his immune system. For the next three months, working with the doctor, Jim found that his health improved significantly. He also made lifestyle changes that supported greater peace of mind and addressed his depression. Although he missed his wife terribly, he found a new volunteer job and began fishing and gardening again. He also began traveling — living near his son in the north each summer and his daughter in the south each winter. Nothing was quite the same, but he found that as long as he stayed well, life was good.

What Happens to Immunity As We Age?

Since the human body produces fewer T cells as it ages, the ability to fight infection often declines. However, the body spontaneously tends to produce more antibodies, which increases our vulnerability to allergies and autoimmune diseases. If T cell levels can be maintained, there is less risk of developing cancer or infection.

Research has shown that nutrition plays a vital role in maintaining this balance in immune capacity. In a recent study on the effects of nutrition and aging, participants were given supplements containing extracts from fruits and vegetables (two capsules of each daily for ninety days). The addition of these supplements to their diet was found to increase their production of T cells and improve immune activity.

Major factors determining the strength of immunity include genetics, inherited tendency to allergies, nutrition, stress, whether you were breast fed, age, the integrity of your digestive system, the health of your microflora, and the presence of infection anywhere in the body. It's encouraging to know that good nutrition can actually affect the way your genetic makeup is expressed. Eating well and including exercise in your schedule can tip the balance toward health.

Rebuilding Immunity

Restoring immunity involves a series of steps that are based on the needs of the individual:

- *Whenever there's an infection, the first priority is to identify and treat it.* In an integrative approach, the doctor may initially prescribe an antibiotic or other medication to clear the infection.
- *Restore good nutrition.* When people become ill and lose their appetite, they may become protein deficient. To support good nutrition, a number of predigested

protein powders can be helpful as supplements including whey or fortified rice protein (see References).

- *Provide basic nutrients.* Sometimes all that is needed is zinc and a good multivitamin (that includes vitamin A and B_6) to restore immunity, since these are key nutrients. However, zinc intake should not exceed 150 mg a day, since excessive levels have been found to depress immunity.

- *Replenish nutritional deficiencies.* Lab tests can be used to measure nutrient levels so that specific deficiencies can be addressed. The levels are later remeasured to be sure they had been restored.

- *Check immune function.* Tests are available to measure T cell and macrophage levels (cellular immunity) and antibody levels (humoral immunity).

- *Enhance depressed immunity.* Herbal and vitamin supplements to improve immune function can be prescribed based on the findings in the lab work. Supplements are targeted to the specific needs of the individual, whether the goal is to stimulate T cells, macrophages, or antibodies.

- *Check hormone levels.* Most people, as they age, experience drops in hormone levels — especially testosterone, adrenal hormones such as DHEA, and growth hormone. Immune function suffers as a result. These hormones can be measured through simple blood tests and then replenished to appropriate levels and monitored periodically through retesting.

❧

Michael Rosenbaum, M.D., of Corte Madera, California, has had an active private practice since 1977 focused on clinical nutrition, immunology, and treatment of allergies. He is a graduate of the Albert Einstein College of Medicine in New York City and holds a master's in clinical biochemistry from the Hebrew University in Jerusalem. He is the author of *SuperSupplements* (Penguin), *Solving the Puzzle of Chronic Fatigue Syndrome* (Life Sciences Press), and numerous articles on nutrition. A frequent presenter to professional medical groups and conferences, he has participated in many television and radio talk shows on the topics of chronic fatigue syndrome, nutrition, and immunity. Dr. Rosenbaum is available for consultations on nutritional therapy, allergy treatment, and antiaging medicine, which can be arranged by calling his office at (415) 927-9450.

CHAPTER THREE

Are You Getting Enough Sleep?

Nancy Faass, M.S.W, M.P.H.

Jean was a busy manager in a large insurance company. The week before annual reports were due, she came down with a nasty flu. Her response was novel and effective — twelve hours of sleep a night. Rather than taking the whole day off, she came to work each day, but only worked until 3:30 in the afternoon. She made it a point to be in bed by 6:00 every night that week. Her energy was good and she was able to keep up with her work schedule (with some intelligent modifications). Although she was tired by the afternoon, the extra sleep enabled Jean to fight the flu successfully and still meet her deadline.

How Much Sleep Do We Need?

Got Sleep?

There is total agreement that sleep is vital to your immunity. Yet we also know that sleep requirements are highly individual and vary greatly from one person to the next. So to stay as healthy as possible, we'll want to find our own ideal balance of sleep, rest, and activity.

For anyone fighting off an illness, it's even more important to get the sleep they really need. Quality sleep has a number of beneficial effects. It obviously provides a chance for the body to rest and repair. In addition, when we're awake and active for a shorter period of time, the body builds up fewer metabolic toxins. Now studies from the National Institutes of Health provide compelling evidence that the immune system doesn't become fully activated for at least $9\frac{1}{2}$ hours of sleep or more.[1]

If you want to enhance your immune response — whether you are fighting off a sudden cold or battling a long-term illness — try extending the hours you sleep until you find yourself waking up naturally, refreshed.[2] If you're really sick, you may need as much as twenty-four hours of bed rest, with as much sleep as possible.

Is Sleep a Question of Life or Death?

Accidents such as the Exxon Valdez oil spill and the nuclear incidents at Chernobyl and Three Mile Island have all been linked to human error — caused by sleep deprivation.[3] At least 100,000 traffic accidents each year are reported to be caused by drowsiness or fatigue — resulting in fatalities to more than 1,500 Americans and injuring another 71,000.[4] In a recent survey from the National Sleep Foundation, nearly one in five drivers reported dozing off at the wheel during the preceding year.[5] Loss of sleep is an issue that affects most of us. The majority of Americans report that they don't get enough sleep:

- *Adults.* Seven in ten say they experience frequent sleep problems.
- *Teenagers.* Almost nine of ten say they need more sleep.[6]
- *Children.* More than two of five have problems falling asleep or feeling fatigued.[7]

We all know sleep is important, but often it's one of the first things we're willing to sacrifice for other priorities. Most of us sense that we're not getting enough rest. But how much is enough? In the 1950s, a massive survey was conducted by the American Cancer Society on the effect of lifestyle on health.[8] More than 1 million Americans were interviewed by volunteers in every county and parish of the U.S. Participants were asked about their exercise, nutrition, smoking, sleep, and other health habits. Seven years later, the survey was repeated. Surveyers compiled data on all the original participants who had died since the first survey. The information was analyzed and reanalyzed to determine the most important lifestyle factors for health and survival. Sleep loss was the factor most closely associated with mortality.

The lowest rates of mortality were for survey participants who said they averaged about eight hours of sleep a night. Studies conducted since that time have had similar findings — eight hours of sleep seems to correlate with good health. The highest death rate at all ages was for those averaging four hours or less sleep a night. A great deal of animal research on sleep deprivation confirms the harmful effects of loss of sleep on health.

Yet currently, more than two-thirds of Americans say they don't get eight hours of sleep a night.[9]

Sleepless in America

In a recent national poll seven of ten Americans say they experience frequent sleep problems, though most have not been diagnosed by a doctor.[10] More than eight out of ten say they would sleep more if they knew they could be healthier. The poll found that one in five adults is so sleepy during the day it interferes with daily activities a few days a week or more.

- *Longer work hours.* Americans are working more and sleeping less. The U.S. labor force is already working longer hours than workers in any industrialized nation in the world — averaging forty-six hours a week on the job. Over one-third work more than fifty hours weekly.[11] As a result, many of us feel pressed for time and stressed.

- *Stress.* Sleep can also be lost due to stress — reflected in symptoms such as worry, fatigue, physical tension, depression, or anxiety.
- *Health problems.* Perhaps the single most important physical issue that interferes with quality sleep is chronic pain, from conditions such as injury, arthritis, ulcers, or headaches. Obstructive sleep apnea, a condition in which breathing is partially obstructed during sleep, is now recognized as more common than previously thought. Diagnosing sleep apnea often requires expert evaluation at a sleep clinic.
- *Nutritional deficiencies.* For example, some people with insomnia appear to have a higher calcium requirement, corrected simply by taking a calcium-magnesium supplement in the evening.

Overall, about half the population is affected by insomnia, according to a nationwide survey.[12] More than half of respondents also reported feeling so sleepy on the job that it affected the quality of their work. Signs of sleep loss in adults include:

- Reduced immunity
- Daytime drowsiness
- Less interest in exercise
- Mood shifts, depression, anxiety, or irritability
- Higher stress
- Impaired memory
- Reduced ability to handle complex tasks or solve problems
- Reduced coordination
- Disorientation
- Increased risk of auto accidents

Barbara had been sick for fifteen years with severe chronic fatigue and fibromyalgia, experiencing frequent pain, depression, and insomnia. She had tried many different approaches, including conventional medicine, Chinese medicine, acupuncture, and homeopathy. She also took supplements and walked for exercise as much as possible. Nothing had resolved the problem.

Treatment also involved balancing her adrenal and hormonal function. Her thyroid had been tested numerous times with normal results each time, so that was initially ruled out. However, her work with a nutritionist revealed other symptoms of thyroid imbalance, so another set of tests were ordered. The lab work indicated that her body wasn't fully converting the thyroid hormones her body produced into a useable form. Once she began taking the thyroid and nutritional supplements, she started sleeping much more normally. Within six weeks, she experienced about an 85 percent improvement in her chronic fatigue syndrome, fibromyalgia, and most of other symptoms. (Case history courtesy of Jeffry Anderson, M.D.)

Sleep Loss and Teenagers

We never really get accustomed to inadequate sleep. Dr. William Dement, director of Stanford's Sleep Disorders Center and a founder of the field of sleep medicine, suggests that most people accumulate a sleep deficit and suffer with the consequences.[13] For teenagers, these include decreases in cognitive functioning and resistance to illness, behavioral abnormalities, and in extreme cases, auto accidents caused by falling asleep while driving.

The best data available on the relationship between teenage sleep and school performance comes from studies in Rhode Island[14] and Minnesota.[15] Researchers in Rhode Island interviewed three thousand high school students in 1998 to document their sleep deficit and relate it to daytime functioning and school performance. In the survey, 87 percent of the students reported that they needed more sleep. Older teens were sleeping less than younger teens. The study found that only 5 percent of parents set bedtimes on school nights. Teenagers who are sleep deprived seem to have symptoms similar to adults — fatigue, moodiness, and lack of alertness. In addition, they may experience:

- Lack of motivation
- Behavioral abnormalities
- Hyperactivity

The study did not show a direct relationship between sleep patterns and grades in school. However, it did find that the students who described themselves as "struggling or failing in school" reported less sleep, irregular schedules, and later bedtimes than students who were getting good grades. Why wasn't there a more direct link between grades and sleep loss? Accumulating sleep debt tends to affect performance over the long term.

One school board in Minnesota performed an experiment to allow students more chance to catch up on sleep by opening schools an hour later.[16] After the first year, 57 percent of teachers reported that students were more alert during the first two periods of the day. An earlier study conducted in Minnesota received even more positive reviews.[17]

Sleep Loss and Schoolchildren

Younger children are also struggling with sleep problems. In a survey of parents in Washington, D.C., almost 11 percent reported that their child had recently had a sleeping disturbance that lasted longer than two weeks.[18] And more than 20 percent of parents said their child took too long to fall asleep, snored, or was fatigued during the day at least once a week.

For young people, eight hours of sleep may not be enough — they may require eight and a half or nine hours of sleep a night — or more.

Signs that children are having sleep problems include all the symptoms seen in adults. Additional signs that may be seen in children include:

- Difficulty falling asleep
- Frequent awakening during the night or insomnia
- Talking during sleep or nightmares
- Difficulty breathing properly
- Bedwetting
- Teeth grinding or clenching

Quality Sleep

When it comes to sleep, quality seems to be as important as quantity. A recent Finnish study has found parallels between good sleep and good health.[19] Researchers surveyed the sleep quality and health status of 1,600 Finnish adults. The survey showed that men with poor quality sleep were more than six times as likely to have poor health. Women who slept poorly were more than three times as likely to have health problems.

The Effect of Sleep Loss

Does it really matter when we lose a little sleep? For more than ten years, studies of animals and humans have been conducted to answer this question. When sleep deprivation is studied, it's describe in terms of sleep debt — essentially sleep loss. Typically animal or human subjects are kept awake for a specific period of time and then their blood is measured for levels of chemical markers such as T cells. The results of animal studies can be applied to humans because sleep functions, body chemistry, and the immune system are quite similar in most mammals. Here is a brief summary of what researchers have found that will help you decide just how important sleep is.

Loss of Five Hours' Sleep in a Single Night

A study at the University of California, San Diego involved health young male volunteers. The loss of just five hours of sleep in one night was found to depress their natural immune responses. There was a 30 percent reduction of infection-fighting T cells — the natural killer cells. An important immune stimulant was also depressed — the cancer-fighting interleukin known as IL-2. After a night of recovery sleep, the T cell activity returned to the original level, but interleukin levels remained depressed. These results suggest the importance of sleep in maintaining immunity and show "that even a modest disturbance of sleep produces a reduction of natural immune responses."[20]

Loss of Four Hours' Sleep a Night, for Six Nights

A study reported in *The Lancet* indicates how sleep loss can affect metabolism. Researchers at the University of Chicago studied physical changes in eleven young men who slept for only four hours a night, six nights in a row.[21] They found that sleep deprivation seemed to trigger a temporary condition that resembled diabetes, which interfered with hormone production and with their ability to metabolize starches and sugars. In response to these and other similar findings, some researchers suggest that extra sleep helps the body keep down excess weight.[22]

Five Days without Sleep

The research on brief sleep deficits has shown a range of effects. In some of the studies, sleep-deprived animals exhibited drops in the levels of protective antibodies. Decreased antibody levels were also found in Norwegian research that monitored men in military training who had gone without sleep for about five days.[23] The most dramatic decreases were in the antibodies that respond to immediate infection — IgM — which dropped by 35 percent. White blood counts also dropped by 30 to 50 percent.

To date, an inconsistent picture emerges from the studies of short-term sleep deficit. Some research has reported depressed levels of immunity, while others found that specific aspects of the immune response actually increased following short-term sleep loss. However, increases in the levels of anti-stress hormones suggest that sleep loss can cause metabolic stress.

No Sleep for Forty Days

Of greatest concern is the evidence found in studies of long-term sleep loss. Sleep deprivation of forty days proved fatal to the animals in research conducted at the National Institute of Mental Health.[24] Autopsies found massive levels of bacteria in the animals' blood and lymph nodes. Dr. Carol Everson and her colleagues concluded that prolonged sleep deprivation appears to cause "a breakdown of host defense against harmful bacteria."[25]

Signs and symptoms that resulted from long-term sleep deprivation included debilitated appearance, skin lesions, wasting syndrome, increased energy expenditure, decreased body temperature during the late stages of deprivation, and increased levels of stress hormones. Four other major abnormalities were also observed:

- Malnutrition
- Decreases in mental function
- Low thyroid levels
- Decreased resistance to infection

Immune activity during sleep seems to maintain balance within the body. It appears that one of the important functions of sleep is to provide the body a time to lower the levels of bacteria in the system.[26] A wide range of yeast and bacteria are normally present in the digestive tract, many of which are beneficial. As long as their levels are kept in balance, they don't present a problem. So sleep seems to provide an opportunity for a kind of internal housekeeping.

The amount of sleep needed is unique to each of us. Research bears this out and also suggests that there is a genetic basis for our sleep requirement. At the University of Texas, researchers monitored behavior and brain waves in two types of rats, and found a consistent difference in sleep patterns from one species to the next.[27] Animal studies at the University of Geneva in Switzerland also found consistent variation. They reported that the study finding "strongly suggests the presence of a gene with a major effect" on the amount of sleep required.[28] This genetic difference was also borne out in research at the University of Helsinki in Finland.[29]

We never get used to doing without sleep. But we all know from personal experience that the body does recovery from loss of sleep. What does it take to recover from sleep debt? Animals suffering sleep loss were allowed to sleep as much as they wanted in the second phase of a study at University of Chicago. Over the course of fifteen days, the majority of the animals showed complete, or almost complete, reversal of symptoms, including improvements in their appearance and energy, and restored balance of thyroid and stress hormones. Researchers reported that "the most prominent features of recovery sleep...were immediate."[30] In some of the animals, the recovery process took longer. This is another example of individual variation.

Getting a Good Night's Sleep

Supporting your immune system through sleep may call for a shift in lifestyle. It could mean letting go of certain pleasures — or trading one pleasure for another. Instead of staying up to watch your favorite show, perhaps record the show on tape. Instead, take a hot shower or luxuriant soak and then settle down for a long, delicious sleep.

Sleep Remedies

If you want to reset your inner clock by encouraging earlier sleep patterns, there are a few remedies that can be helpful. Before using an herbal or nutritional remedy, and if you have a health condition or are taking medication, be sure to check with your health-care practitioner as appropriate. The safest approach is to start with minimal doses — for example, taking only one capsule per day for the first three days. When it is clear that the remedy agrees with your system, gradually increase it to the recommended dose. Avoid making other changes during that time, so that if there is a problem, the cause will be apparent.

Napping

Does a nap make up for sleep lost at night? There is also good evidence that naps are beneficial based on a number of studies, including those conducted at the Henry Ford Hospital in Detroit. Napping has been found "clearly beneficial to someone who is a normal sleeper but who is getting insufficient sleep at night. . . . We don't understand the underlying neurobiology, but sleep time is cumulative. A two-hour or a four-hour nap, before [staying] up all night, does provide additional alertness the next day." NASA research found similar results.[31] However, it is important not to nap too close to bedtime, which could interrupt your basic sleep pattern.

Insomnia

Insomnia that continues for more than three months is best addressed by a physician or by sleep experts. There are now sleep centers located throughout the U.S., listed in *The Promise of Sleep,* by Dr. William Dement.[32]

Rest and Sleep

There is a major difference between resting in bed and sleeping. Sleep that allows for a deeper resting state is especially important, because it offers the opportunity to bring metabolic restoration to the body, on a level that doesn't seem to occur from rest alone.[33] We know from recent research that an extended period of sleep is required for the immune system to become fully engaged, which may be the reason why we usually sleep so much longer when we are ill.[34] Research also suggests that deep sleep allows more antibody production.

Sleep and Immunity

Experience and common sense suggest that sleep is helpful when we're sick. We also see this wisdom in animals, who may sleep for as long as a week when they are sick or injured. From the viewpoint of science, research has also demonstrated the essential role of sleep in promoting immunity. Given all this evidence, the greatest challenge may simply be acting on that wisdom. That means finding ways to fit sleep into our hectic lives. Sweet dreams.

In short:
- For young people, the amount of sleep needed appears to be more than eight hours — eight and a half, nine, or more hours a night.
- When we're ill, we apparently need as much as nine and a half hours' sleep a night or even much more, according to NIH research. (For more on this topic, see *Lights Out* by T. S. Wiley with Bent Formby.)
- One good way to find out how much sleep one needs is to go to bed at the same time each night and notice what time you naturally wake up without an alarm.
- What is the best sleep cycle? Depending on your own makeup, you may also need to go to bed early in order to wake up refreshed. So if you still awaken feeling tired after a full night's sleep, gradually move your bedtime earlier until you wake up naturally, well rested. You may even find yourself slightly disoriented for a few days while your body adjusts to your new sleep schedule.
- It can take as much as two weeks to really catch up on sleep if you have a sleep deficit.

Nancy Faass, M.S.W., M.P.H., is a writer and editor in San Francisco who provides book and project development in integrative medicine and the social sciences. Ms. Faass is developer and editor of *Integrating Complementary Medicine into Health Systems.* She is also codeveloper and coeditor of *Optimal Digestion* from HarperCollins with Trent Nichols, M.D.

Notes

1. T. S. Wiley with B. Formby, *Lights Out* (New York: Pocket Books, 2000).
2. C. Hublin, J. Kaprio, M. Partinen et al., "Insufficient Sleep: A Population-Based Study in Adults," *Sleep* 24, no. 4 (June 2001): 392–400.
3. S. Coren, *Sleep Thieves: An Eye-Opening Exploration into the Science and Mysteries of Sleep* (New York: Free Press/Simon & Schuster, 1996).
4. National Highway Traffic Safety Administration (NHTSA), 1994. Website www.counseling.caltech.edu/html/sleep.html, accessed May 2001.
5. W B & A Market Research, *2001 Sleep in America Poll* (Washington, D.C.: National Sleep Foundation, 2001). Website www.sleepfoundation.org, accessed May 2001.
6. Montgomery County Public Schools, Rockville, Maryland, "Article on Teen Sleep Deprivation." Website www.mcps.k12.md.us/schools/bcchs/info/ptsa/sleep.html, accessed May 2001.
7. Reuters Health, "Sleep Troubles Common Among Schoolchildren," April 2, 2001, www.reutershealth.com/archive/2001/04/02/links/20010402elin016.html.
8. W. C., Dement, M.D., *The Promise of Sleep* (New York: Dell, 1999).
9. See note 5 above.
10. See note 5 above.
11. L. D. Hatfield, "America's Bedroom Blues," *San Francisco Chronicle,* March 28, 2001.
12. See note 5 above.
13. See note 8 above.
14. See note 6 above.
15. Minneapolis School District Trial, 1998. Website www.mcps.k12.md.us/schools/bcchs/info/ptsa/sleep.html, accessed May 2001. Final report available at www.carei.coled.umn.edu. Also, see CNN Networks, *Sleep Well, Do Well,* February 27, 2001. Website www1.cnn.com/2001/HEALTH/parenting/02/27/kids.sleep/.
16. See note 15 above.
17. See note 15 above.
18. See note 7 above.
19. See note 2 above.
20. M. Irwin, J. McClintock, C. Costlow et al., "Partial Night Sleep Deprivation Reduces Natural Killer and Cellular Immune Responses in

Humans," *Federation of American Societies for Experimental Biology Journal* 10, no. 5 (April 1996): 643–53.

21. K. Spiegel, R. Leproult, E. Van Cauter, "Impact of Sleep Debt on Metabolic and Endocrine Function," *The Lancet* 354, no. 9188 (October 1999): 1435–39.

22. See note 1 above.

23. A. Boyum, P. Wiik, E. Gustavsson et al., "The Effect of Strenuous Exercise, Calorie Deficiency and Sleep Deprivation on White Blood Cells, Plasma Immunoglobulins and Cytokines," *Scandinavian Journal of Immunology* 43, no. 2 (February 1996): 228–35.

24. C. A. Everson and L. A. Toth, "Systemic Bacterial Invasion Induced by Sleep Deprivation," *American Journal of Physiology* 278, no. 4 (April 2000): R905–16.

25. See note 24 above.

26. M. Rosenbaum, "Immunity against Invaders." In T. Nichols and N. Faass, eds., *Optimal Digestion* (New York: HarperCollins, 1999). Also, see note 1 above.

27. M. R. Opp, "Rat Strain Differences Suggest a Role for Corticotropin-Releasing Hormone in Modulating Sleep," *Physiology and Behavior* 63, no. 1 (December 1997): 67–74.

28. P. Franken, A. Malafosse, and M. Tafti, "Genetic Variation in EEG Activity during Sleep in Inbred Mice," *American Journal of Physiology* 275, no. 4, pt. 2 (October 1998): R1127–37.

29. I. Hilakivi and T. Taira, "Strain Difference in Early Postnatal Sleep-Wake Behavior between Alko Alcohol and Wistar Rats," *Acta Physiologica Scandinavia* 154, no. 1 (May 1995): 75–80.

30. C. A. Everson, M. A. Gilliland, C. A. Kushida et al., "Sleep Deprivation in the Rat: IX. Recovery," *Sleep* 12, no. 1 (February 1989): 60–67.

31. See note 8 above.

32. See note 8 above.

33. Len Saputo, M.D., written communication, June 7, 2001.

34. See note 1 above.

CHAPTER FOUR

What about Water?

Nancy Faass, M.S.W, M.P.H.

As a child, Jason never felt thirsty. In fact, he didn't even like the taste of water. Several times a day, his mother would feed him a little water on a spoon, but soon he would push it away in frustration. In the summer, he was healthier and more active, so it didn't seem to matter. But as soon as cold weather set in, he began cycling through colds and flus that lasted about six months of every year.

It was not until he was a young man that it was discovered he might be missing a vital brain chemical that carries thirst messages to the body. Doctors have found that in such cases, the answer is simply to take fluids on a regular schedule. Gradually, Jason overcame his dislike for water. Every day he carries two bottles of water with his lunch, one for midmorning and the other for midafternoon. The benefits of the water would be difficult to prove, but it's interesting to know that he hardly ever gets sick.

We can only survive a week without water, whereas we can live as long as six weeks without food. What are the vital links between our fluid intake and our immunity?

Water carries away waste and toxins from our cells and from the entire body. Some toxins are actually by-products of our own metabolism and our immune function. Some are manufactured by bacteria and other microbes. In addition, toxins are introduced from natural or industrial sources through food, water, and air. Fortunately, water washes many of these toxins out of the body.

Water replenishes the systems that cleanse the body — the blood and lymph, which are primarily water. The lymph is a system of fluid laden with antibodies (our immune artillery) and white blood cells. This system has been recognized for thousands of years as a source of purification — the Romans named it lymph, which means "clear spring water."[1] It is likely that this cleansing process helps to keep bacteria in balance. Although many of the bacteria in our body are beneficial, to stay healthy, we need to maintain that balance.

Are You Getting Enough Water?

Our bodies are about 70 percent water: ten to twelve gallons.[2] We know that every cell in our body requires water to function — to bring in nourishment and to carry away toxins. When these functions can't be performed because of dehydration, a range of symptoms can occur.[3]

- *At 1 percent dehydration,* most people get very thirsty, which is the body's warning sign that we need more liquids.

  By the time we experience thirst, we're already beginning to dehydrate. People who have no natural thirst have no warning that they're becoming dehydrated.

- *A 2 to 5 percent dehydration* can cause dry mouth, flushed skin, fatigue, headache, or impaired physical performance. We know that as the body becomes more dehydrated, there is less inclination toward exercise. Chronic, low-grade dehydration may sneak up on us. At this stage, signs of dehydration include:

* Headache, which occurs as toxins begin building up in the body
* Poor digestion or constipation
* Urine that is scant and darker in color
* Extremely dry or itchy skin
* Fatigue
* Lapses in concentration

- *A 6 to 8 percent dehydration* can increase body temperature, the rate of breathing, and pulse. We may have fairly dramatic symptoms if we dehydrate rapidly on a hot day or after intense exercise, experiencing:

    * Dizziness, fainting, or nausea
    * Sudden weakness, fatigue, or muscle cramps
    * Labored breathing from exertion

- *A 10 to 11 percent dehydration* can result in muscle spasms or delirium and may lead to poor blood circulation and even failing kidney function. A 15 percent dehydration can be fatal.

If you've experienced any of those symptoms and you drink less than six glasses of water a day, monitor your water intake. Then try gradually increasing the amount of water you drink until you're having six to eight cups. Then notice if your health has improved.

Most of these symptoms are so common that they could be caused by any number of health conditions. This makes it difficult to determine what the underlying problem really is. But getting enough fluid is an important aspect of good health. Unfortunately, there is limited research on the link between immunity and dehydration. However, it is clear that some people with chronic dehydration tend to be sick more often, plagued by frequent colds, flu, or other types of health issues.

Why Water Matters

In our bodies, water is the medium through which everything occurs. Water transports nutrients and oxygen. It is essential for the digestion of proteins and fats and plays a vital role in the actual production of energy. Water also has very specific functions — regulating body temperature by insulating against both heat and cold. It lubricates and cushions the eyes, brain, and spinal cord as well as the joints and vital organs. It moistens and purifies our skin and the oxygen we breathe.[3,4]

The Body Is Mostly Water

- Blood is 83 percent water.
- The brain is 75 percent water.
- Muscle is 73 percent water.
- Fat is 25 percent water.
- Bone is 22 percent water.

How Much Water Is Enough?

Americans are doing better about drinking water — on average about six cups of water a day, according to a survey taken in 2000.[5] That's up from 4.6 cups of water a day in 1998. Yet many Americans claim to experience frequent health problems, including fatigue and grogginess, that can be caused by dehydration. A recent survey found that:

- Only a third report drinking eight or more glasses of water a day.
- Almost a third drink three or fewer glasses.
- Almost 10 percent say they don't drink water at all.

We often hear physicians recommend that we drink six to eight glasses of water a day. A study performed in the Netherlands found that healthy elderly people surveyed drink on average just under nine cups of water a day.[6] Some of us actually need more, so it's equally important to determine your own level. Like every other aspect of body chemistry, there is typically a personal balance point for each person.

What is your ideal level of water intake? Factor in your physical size, your body type, the climate you live in, and how active you are. It's also important to know whether you require extra liquid intake because of a special health condition (for example, a tendency to have kidney stones). On the other hand, if you take certain medications, it could be important not to drink too much liquid. Other determining factors include how many dehydrating beverages you drink, like caffeine or alcohol.

What to Drink

What are the best fluids to drink? According to the Human Nutrition Center at Rockefeller University, water is the "best choice for proper hydration."[7]

Spring water is one of the best options. Bottled waters also include glacial and mineral waters from across the globe, including Canada, the French Alps, Fiji, Iceland, and Italy. Other good water sources are bottled or tap water that's well filtered, using a method such as carbon-block or reverse-osmosis filtration. Use bottled or filtered water in cooking, to make herb teas, and to dilute fresh fruit or vegetable juices. See the table on page 50 for information on the advantages of various filtration systems.[8]

What if water tastes bad to you? Some people find that they don't enjoy drinking water. In a recent consumer survey, 13 percent said they didn't like the taste of water, and 12 percent said they preferred other beverages. For both these issues, the answer may be to find a type of water that is compatible, such as imported waters or lightly flavored drinks. Adding some minimal flavoring to the water can make it much easier to drink an adequate amount.

- Experiment to find the products that taste best to you.
- Taste test the wide variety of bottled and mineral waters.

- Flavor water with a slice or two of lemon or lime.
- Add an herbal tea bag to water that is room temperature, hot, or cooled.
- Boost the nutrient content of water with a powdered supplement such as Emergen-C or Ola Loa.
- Try lightly flavored waters such as Fruit Water, now available for those making the transition to water from juice or other sweeter beverages.
- Make fresh fruit juices (diluted about half and half with water).
- Try any of the light juices such as Wellness Water or other products. Check the carbohydrate content on the label to be sure they don't contain too much added sweetener.
- Iced or very cold drinks are best avoided, according to traditional Chinese medicine, because of the possible effect of extreme temperatures on the stomach.
- Enjoy warm or hot drinks including herbal tea, green tea, or chai; hot water with warming herbs such as cinnamon and cardamom; ginger tea; lemon water; or vegetable broth.
- Hot water is considered a universal tonic throughout Asia and an effective remedy for many illnesses. A healthy morning ritual begins with first drinking something warm, often simply plain hot water. This prepares the stomach, just as a hot shower is invigorating and gets the blood moving. Sipping hot (but not scalding) water throughout the day is also considered very beneficial to health and is believed to maintain or restore digestion.[9]

Increasing Your Water Intake

Drinking water can become a habit. Times of day that are particularly good for drinking water include first thing in the morning, when you get up, midmorning, and midafternoon. The British take a break in the late afternoon for a fortifying cup of tea and perhaps something light to eat. A number of other pleasant rituals can be adapted to your lifestyle. One approach is to take a large sip of water every thirty minutes and to drink a whole glass of water twenty to thirty minutes before eating your meals.[10]

1. *Getting enough water to drink.* The most frequent reason given by Americans for not drinking water is lack of time, reported by 21 percent in a recent survey.[11] Another 18 percent reported that they forget to drink water, don't have good water available, or can't leave their desks for a break. Many of these problems could be resolved by carrying bottled water or a favorite beverage to work.

2. *What if you never get thirsty?* In a nationwide survey, 8 percent reported that they never feel thirsty.[12] In another study, 10 percent reported that they never drank water. One of the best ways to cope with lack of thirst is to drink water on schedule. Make sure that it's a pleasant experience, something you look forward to. That means finding beverages you really like and identifying the times of day when you can realistically have something healthy to drink. It may also involve some extra logistics, like buying a handsome ceramic, no-spill mug for your desk or a beverage holder for your car. Again, if there's no water cooler or filter at work, it also means bringing the bottled water you need with you each day.

3. *Drinking liquids in the evening.* Bedtime is not always the best time to drink water.[13] It has been documented that drinking water mostly before 6:00 P.M. can reduce the likelihood of nocturnal bathroom visits. Those who do not have this problem may find that the evening is a good time to fit in another glass of water, while they're reading, watching television, or relaxing.

Other Beverages

There are an endless number of products on the market that taste good and are thirst quenching. The key is to become as conscientious about reading the labels on your beverages as you are on food items. First check the carbohydrate content for the amount of added sweeteners, such as sugar, corn syrup, fructose, glucose, honey, maple syrup, fruit juice concentrate, or other additives that tend to promote weight gain when consumed in excess. Also check the level of caffeine and other chemicals and food additives. If the beverage dehydrating, like coffee and alcohol, moderation is the solution.

Fruit juice. Bottled fruit juices are usually highly processed. The juice is cooked (pasteurized), bottled, and shipped, so the inevitable destruction of vitamins and enzymes has taken place. What remains is the fruit sugar — fructose — which tastes good but has certain drawbacks.[14] A quart of orange juice, for example, contains the juice of ten oranges. We would almost never sit down and eat ten oranges, but we think nothing of drinking a pint or even a quart of juice. With juice or soda, check for the carbohydrate content and sugars so you will know how sweet they really are.[15] A good way around this is to eat fresh fruit rather than drinking the juice.

Sodas. Carbonated beverages are high in phosphoric acid, which contributes to osteoporosis — the loss of calcium and other minerals in the bones.[16] They may also contain caffeine, artificial sweeteners, and other additives. Although artificial sweeteners prevent weight gain, the research on most of these products has shown mixed results. As a treat, drinking soda with artificial sweeteners is probably not a problem. The issue becomes how often they're consumed — weekly, daily, or hourly?

In general, the craving for sweets can be cut by drinking more water and other lighter drinks. Cravings can also be minimized by taking buffered vitamin C or a chromium supplement.[17] If you find that your consumption of fruit, fruit juice, or sodas is excessive, make an effort to identify and eliminate the underlying cause through a resource such as *The Diet Cure* by Julia Ross.

Dehydrating Beverages

We tend to forget that hydrating and dehydrating beverages tend to cancel each other out. Hydrating beverages serve to promote appropriate water retention, the basis for healthy functioning. Healthful beverages that keep your body hydrated include water, juice, milk, and herbal teas. Carbonated sodas without caffeine aren't dehydrating, but they are often heavily sweetened.

Although Americans typically drink about eight servings of hydrating beverages each day, they also have about five servings of dehydrating beverages daily.[18] The most popular dehydrating beverages are coffee, tea, carbonated soda with caffeine, beer, wine, and other alcoholic drinks. Of these drinks, alcohol seems to be the most dehydrating. Beverages that dehydrate act as mild diuretics, increasing urine production and loss of fluid from the body. They don't provide as much hydration to the body as hydrating beverages do. When we drink coffee, tea, caffeinated soda, and alcoholic drinks, we're not getting the same hydrating benefit as when we drink pure water.

Coffee. In moderation, most foods and beverages don't pose a significant problem. A cup of coffee a day is not a problem for most people.[19] If what you're looking for is a morning pick-me-up, try adding some form of protein to your breakfast (such as a smoothie) and carry snacks that include some protein (like nuts) for later in the day. If coffee is just another beverage to you, try switching over to spring or mineral waters. If coffee or tea drinking is a social ritual, moderate your intake by drinking herb tea or green tea.[20] When you want to break the habit, you may try lowering your coffee intake gradually by switching over to lattes or cappuccinos.

Alcoholic beverages. The research on drinking alcohol is mixed.[21] Here, too, use discretion. Researchers found lower rates of heart disease among the French, associated with the intake of red wine.[22] In the United States, some studies have also found that moderate intake of alcoholic beverages is linked to increased relaxation and greater longevity. Although one or two glasses of wine a day have beneficial effects, they come at a price. It is well documented that alcoholic beverages have toxic effects on the liver and nervous system. They are linked to cancer and can be addictive.[23] Since alcoholic beverages are also dehydrating, they have to be subtracted from your total water intake. Drink eight ounces of water for every alcoholic beverage you drink.[24]

Clean Drinking Water

Type of Water or Filter	Advantages	Disadvantages
Tap water To check the quality of your tap water, call your water district; useful information can be found on the Web at www.ewg.org.	Inexpensive and available; quality varies. Boil for fifteen to twenty minutes to remove chlorine, bacteria, and some parasites, especially if you are immune compromised.	Quality varies. Can contain chlorine, fluoride, heavy metals, THMs (trihalomethanes), cryptosporidium, giardia, and other parasites and their cysts.

Clean Drinking Water (continued)		
Type of Water or Filter	Advantages	Disadvantages
Bottled Water When ordering bottled water delivery, request testing information; inquire about the source of the water — is it natural spring, distilled, or filtered municipal water? — and read labels.	Usually tested and prefiltered; spring water may be a good natural source of minerals.	Soft and even hard plastic containers outgas toxic compounds including plastisizers (phthalates), vinyl chloride, and bisphenol-A (an endocrine-disrupter). Glass containers are best.
Ceramic Carbon Filters Two-step filtration provided by compacted activated carbon and porous ceramic.	Removes most bacteria, parasites, and cysts; chemicals such as chlorine, pesticides, most solvents, and some radioactive pollutants; some heavy metals; sediment.	Doesn't remove fluoride or certain heavy metals, viruses, or other very small microbes.
Carbon Block Filter Check manufacturer's specifications.	Removes chlorine, pesticides, and solvents; some radioactive contaminants.	Doesn't remove bacteria, asbestos, fluoride, heavy metals, or some radioactive compounds.

Clean Drinking Water (continued)		
Type of Water or Filter	Advantages	Disadvantages
Mechanical Filter Some are impregnated with silver compounds.	Filters out debris, bacteria, large parasites, and cysts down to 1 or 0.5 microns; also kills some bacteria.	Does not remove asbestos, chlorine, fluoride, heavy metals, THMs, or most volatile chemicals such as solvents or pesticides.
Reverse-Osmosis Filter Exceptionally thorough multistage water filtration that includes membrane and carbon filters.	Removes almost everything, except pesticides, radon, and volatile organic chemicals; to compensate, many systems come with add-on carbon filtration units. The two in combination provide the most thorough filtration available.	Also removes good minerals and renders water "lifeless"; may be supplemented with a unit to add minerals back in; requires periodic filter change or back-flushing with chlorine; can outgas plastic compounds into water, requiring an additional filtration step.
Granulated, Activated Charcoal Typically comes in small pitcher-style filters, faucet filters, and some prefilters.	Better than drinking unfiltered water; removes some chemicals and particulates, including chlorine, mercury, THMs, and large parasites.	Doesn't remove bacteria or protozoa under 4 microns in size or asbestos, fluoride, certain heavy metals, or most radioactive compounds.

Clean Drinking Water (continued)		
Type of Water or Filter	Advantages	Disadvantages
Alkaline Water With granulated activated charcoal prefilter (impregnated with silver); can be linked to carbon block for additional filtration.	May restore normal acid-base balance in the body and aid detoxification; the unit can be linked to another filtration system as a prefilter.	Same limitations as other granulated charcoal filters; best in combination with prefilter; misses chemicals, fluoride, heavy metals, and viruses.

Source: In Jeffry Anderson, M.D., "Avoid Toxic Exposure." T. Nichols, M.D. and N. Faass. *Optimal Digestion.* New York: HarperCollins, 1999.

When We Need Extra Water

In some circumstances we need to drink even more water than usual.

To fight off infections such as a cold or the flu, increasing water intake will help the lymph system wash away germs and their toxins. Drink more fluids if you've been vomiting or have had diarrhea; try something soothing like peppermint, chamomile, or a combination of the two such as Sleepytime Tea.

With certain medications, it's important not to drink too much water. With others, you may need to drink additional fluids. Learn about the medications you are taking that might affect your hydration. Make sure you have all the facts.[25]

Before and during exercise, drink fluids and particularly water, to reduce body temperature, moderate cardiovascular stress, and improve performance. After a strenuous workout, it's important to replace the fluids you've lost.[26]

Water and Weight Loss

For those trying to lose weight, water is twice as beneficial as other beverages, because it doesn't contain the sweeteners, high calories, and carbohydrates found in sodas and sports drinks. To verify the content of your beverages, just read the information on carbohydrates and sugars on the label of your favorite quencher. Drinks containing artificial sweeteners are not recommended.[27] Water and light drinks also tend to cut food cravings — try this for yourself.

Replacing Fluids During Sports Events

1. Plain water is best for exercise that lasts an hour or less.
2. Don't depend on thirst. Drink before you get thirsty.
3. Drink water before a sporting event or physical activity. Two cups of water about two hours before an event is about right.
4. Sip water during an event ($\frac{1}{3}$ to $\frac{3}{4}$ cup every ten to twenty minutes).
5. Weigh in before and after a sporting event or heavy work-out. After the event replace fluids with two cups of water for every one pound lost.

The American College of Sports Medicine recommends that for exercise events lasting more than an hour, "consider the addition of carbohydrates and/or electrolytes to a fluid replacement solution...containing 4 percent to 8 percent carbohydrates."[28]

Pregnancy and Water Intake

A number of common complaints of pregnancy can be addressed by drinking sufficient water during pregnancy — these include constipation, water retention, bloating, bladder infections, and hemorrhoids. Extreme dehydration can result in reduced amounts of amniotic fluid and can even be a factor in premature or difficult labor. An important way to help minimize these pregnancy-related maladies is to drink plenty of water. Water carries nutrients through the blood to the baby and is vital in maintaining good health during pregnancy. Experts recommend that pregnant women drink eight to ten eight-ounce glasses of water daily — and one extra glass for each hour of physical activity. Sufficient hydration can make the experience of pregnancy healthier and more enjoyable for both mother and baby.

Children and Fluid Intake

It is also important that children get enough fluids. They are less equipped to handle high temperatures than adults, because they have less sweating capacity. Therefore, in the heat, they need to drink even more water than adults do. An added benefit of giving a child water or light drinks instead of lots of juice or soda is that the potential for childhood obesity may be reduced.

When infants and young children are ill, frequent vomiting and severe diarrhea can quickly lead to dehydration. Weak rice water can be given to children with upset digestion. Fluid replacement is best done with water that contains electrolytes — minerals, a little salt, and a little sweetener — to retain the proper fluid balance. Electrolytes can be purchased as products like Gatorade or little packets of electrolyte minerals from the health food store. You can also make an electrolyte solution at home:

1 quart of drinking water or boiled water

2 Tbsp. honey or sugar

$\frac{1}{4}$ tsp. sea salt or table salt

$\frac{1}{4}$ tsp. baking soda (bicarbonate of soda)

Optional: $\frac{1}{2}$ cup of orange juice can be added to increase
the potassium content.[29]

Getting Your Child to Drink Enough Water

- Over time, encourage your child to try a number of the light drinks we've described here. For children without thirst, these drinks seem to make the greatest difference in whether they actually drink enough fluid daily. Good choices include:

  Fresh juice or half juice and half spring water
  Light bottled drinks such as Fruit Water or light juices
  Simple homemade soups
  Flavorful, nourishing blender drinks
  Herbal teas free of caffeine
  Light soy beverages

- Be sure not to overdo your child's intake of carbohydrates with too much fruit, fruit juice, sweet vegetables like carrots, or the numerous sweeteners found even in apparently nutritious products. Monitor carbohydrate intake by reading labels.

- Encourage your child to form the habit of drinking water or something light first thing in the morning and, if possible, an hour before breakfast and dinner.

- Use colorful, interesting cups, sports bottles, and straws to help pique their interest in drinking more.

- On hot days, keep the water cool but not cold.

- When you shop, make good choices. Do not stock the fridge with a lot of tempting sugar- and caffeine-filled drinks that could derail your efforts.

- Set a good example by drinking plenty of water and fluids too!

Dehydration and Aging

As we age, our thirst decreases. Perhaps as a result, dehydration, which can sometimes even be fatal, is one of the most frequent causes of hospitalization in people over age sixty-five. Aging is also associated with lower levels of total body fluids, reduced fitness level, and decreased kidney function — all of which can contribute to dehydration. It's possible to make up for the subtle loss of function that happens as part of the natural aging process by drinking extra fluid to keep the body detoxified. Water can be considered a fountain of youth as we age.

Drinking Water and Travel

While traveling in the United States, drink bottled water rather than tap water. For example, Milwaukee, Wisconsin, had a cryptosporidium (microscopic parasite) outbreak spread through tap water that required hospitalization for thousands and killed more than one hundred people.[30] Drinking fountains in Yosemite National Park have been found to harbor potentially harmful microbes such as giardia.[31] When traveling overseas, make it a point to educate yourself about whether quality bottled water will be available and carry iodine tablets, particularly if you will be in a developing country. Worldwide, waterborne infectious disease such as typhoid and cholera are the second leading cause of death, accounting for more than five million fatalities a year.[32]

How Important Is Water to Our Health?

Although we don't yet have the in-depth research we need to draw clear conclusions, doctors have observed a link between drinking sufficient water and good health.[33] Why haven't we heard more about the importance of water drinking? Research is expensive. Like the air we breathe, water can't be patented. As a result, lifestyle factors tend to be less well researched.

Conditions that may be improved by drinking sufficient water include:

- Hyperacidity
- Constipation
- Mild mood swings

- Kidney stones. Anyone with a history of kidney stones may benefit from sufficient water intake, because water dissolves calcium in the urine, reducing the risk of stone formation. Among physicians, urologists are probably most likely to extol the virtues of water.
- Urinary tract infections. For men and for women, these may be prevented by drinking enough water.

You can observe the effects of drinking water on your own health. Just be sure to proceed gradually. Consider taking electrolyte capsules if your water intake exceeds eight cups a day. Check with your doctor about what's right for you. Enjoy.

Safe Water Tips

1. Avoid drinking tap water as your main source of drinking water, especially water containing chlorine and fluoride.
2. Drink either bottled water or filtered water, depending on your family's needs and budget.
3. Consider having your regular drinking water professionally assessed, particularly if you have a well.
4. If you must drink tap water, avoid the first morning's water and boil it for twenty minutes.
5. Avoid using tap water in baby formulas and young children's foods. Never use hot tap water, which may contain even more lead and higher levels of bacteria.
6. If you shower regularly with chlorinated water, invest in an inexpensive dechlorinator and filter attachment for the shower. (See the resources section.)
7. When traveling, be extra careful about contaminated water. When camping, boil your water for fifteen to twenty minutes, use iodine tablets, or use an appropriate travel filtration system with a very fine filter.
8. Read up on drinking water issues in sources such as

> *Save Our Planet* by Diane MacEachern and *Healthy Water for a Longer Life* by Martin Fox.
>
> Courtesy: Elson Haas, M.D. *The Staying Healthy Shopper's Guide* (Berkeley, Calif.: Celestial Arts Press, 1999).

⚬

Nancy Faass, M.S.W., M.P.H., is a writer and editor in San Francisco who provides book and project development in integrative medicine and the social sciences. With a master's degree in public health from the University of California at Berkeley and a master's in social work from Catholic University in Washington, D.C., she has worked as a science editor at U.C.S.F., as an archivist, and in scholarly publishing. She has served as a program coordinator in both social services and in education. Ms. Faass is developer and editor of *Integrating Complementary Medicine into Health Systems.* She is also codeveloper and coeditor of *Optimal Digestion* from HarperCollins with Trent Nichols, M.D.

Notes

1. American Dietetic Association. Website www.eatright.org/olderamericans/waterhydration.html, accessed April 14, 2001.
2. R. Larson-Duyff, *The American Dietetic Association's Complete Food and Nutrition Guide* (New York: Wiley, 1998).
3. B. Levine, "Oral Comments on the Report of the 2000 Dietary Guidelines Advisory Committee," International Bottled Water Association. Website www.incongress.com/issues/article.cfm, accessed April 5, 2001.
4. B. Carey, "Hard to Swallow: Do You Really Need Eight Glasses of Water Every Day?" *Los Angeles Times,* November 20, 2000, p. S1.
5. See note 3 above.
6. W. C. Bastiaansen and L. A. Kroot, "Fluid Intake by Healthy Old People: A Literature Survey," *Tijdschrift voor Gerontologie en Geriatrie* 31, no. 1 (February 2000): 27–30.

7. L. Keegan and G. T. Keegan, M.D., *Healing Waters* (New York: Berkeley Books, 1998).

8. S.V. Anderson, M.D., "The Basics." In T. Nichols, and N. Faass, eds. *Optimal Digestion* (New York: HarperCollins, 1999) and Jeffry Anderson, M.D., written communication, May 2, 2001.

9. E. Korngold, "Chinese Medicine and Digestion." In T. Nichols. M.D., and N. Faass, eds. *Optimal Digestion* (New York: HarperCollins, 1999).

10. E. Cutler, M.D., written communication, April 27, 2001.

11. International Bottled Water Association, "Survey: America's Poor Drinking Habits Contradict Knowledge of Health Risks," 2001. Website www.bottled water.org/public/InfoForRepNatFactSheettest.html, accessed May 7, 2001.

12. See note 11 above.

13. See note 7 above.

14. See note 8 above.

15. P. Lynn, M.D., written communication, May 12, 1999.

16. See note 8 above.

17. J. Stine, nutritional consultant, oral communication, August 6, 2001.

18. See note 4 above.

19. L. Saputo, M.D., oral communication, July 2, 2001.

20. See note 8 above.

21. See note 19 above.

22. S. Rotondo, A. di Castelnuovo, and G. de Gaetano, "The Relationship between Wine Consumption and Cardiovascular Risk: From Epidemiological Evidence to Biological Plausibility," *Italian Heart Journal* 2, no. 1 (January 2001): 1–8.

23. See note 19 above.

24. See note 8 above.

25. Website www.sparklingspring.com/waterhealth.html#dehydration, accessed May 14, 2001.

26. V. A. Convertino, L. E. Armstrong, E. F. Coyle et al., "American College of Sports Medicine Position Stand: Exercise and Fluid Replacement," *Medicine and Science in Sports and Exercise* 28, no. 1 (January 1996): i–vii.

27. See note 8 above.

28. See note 26 above.

29. See note 7 above.

30. A. C. McDonald, W. R. MacKenzie, D. G. Addiss et al., "Cryptosporidium Parvum-Specific Antibody Responses among Children Residing in Milwaukee during the 1993 Waterborne Outbreak," *Journal of Infectious Diseases* 189, no. 8 (May 2001): 1373–79.

31. T. P. Welch, "Risk of Giardiasis from Consumption of Wilderness Water in

North America: A Systematic Review of Epidemiologic Data," *Internal Journal of Infectious Diseases* 4, no. 2 (2000): 100–3.

32. K. C. Carroll and L. Reimer, "Infectious Diarrhea: Pathogens and Treatment," *The Lebanese Medical Journal* 48, no. 4 (July–August 2000): 270–77.

33. E. Haas, M.D., *The Staying Healthy Shopper's Guide* (Berkeley, Calif.: Celestial Arts Press, 1999). Also see notes 8, 9, 10, 11, 19, and 30.

CHAPTER FIVE

Getting Your Immune System in Shape

Roger Jahnke, O.M.D.

Tim first came to the clinic as a patient seeking acupuncture and support in his struggle with HIV. He participated in the Circle of Life group we ran for people with chronic illness, which focused on optimizing lifestyle. He also came to our Qigong classes. When Tim dropped out of sight, I assumed we might not see him again. This was in the early years of the AIDS epidemic, and most of the people we saw who had HIV were dying quite young.

Five or six years later, I met Tim again when I was teaching a Qigong class in San Francisco at a conference. Although he looked very familiar, I couldn't place him at first, this tall slender man in the back row. After the class, he introduced himself. Tim was not only surviving HIV; he exuded radiant health. His job required him to travel extensively, yet everywhere he had lived he made it a point to get involved in a support group and a Qigong class. He felt that these two factors had been instrumental in promoting his good health.

You've probably noticed that there's a healing side to exercise: It can chase the blues, help fight stress, and raise your energy. But when is exercise actually therapeutic?

Millennia ago, the people of ancient China and India developed methods of exercise with exceptional healing effects. Although they evolved continents apart, Qigong, t'ai chi, and yoga have certain similarities. They can all be described as meditative exercise and all involve:

- Relaxation and concentration
- A focus on the breath
- Gradual, purposeful movement

We know from modern research that these disciplines have been found to promote the effectiveness of the immune system. They were used purposefully in ancient cultures as a complement to medical treatment.

Qigong is still valued in traditional Chinese medicine and today is practiced throughout China by millions. Each morning, the parks there are filled with people performing Qigong and t'ai chi (a form of Qigong). These exercises are also used in hospitals and sanitariums as part of the therapy for people suffering from conditions such as cancer and tuberculosis. In Indian Ayurvedic medicine, lifestyle is an integral part of treatment. Specific exercises may be prescribed for individual patients, based on their condition and body type.

The Scientific Evidence

The research is clear on two points: that oxygen deficiency leads to decreased immune function and that moderate amounts of mild exercise can increase immune function. Self-healing, self-regulation, and self-repair tend to be stimulated and maximized through simple and meditative exercise movement and breathing. Some of these benefits include:

- *Increased oxygen.* In essence, these practices provide a kind of tune-up to your metabolism. But unlike vigorous exercise, Qigong and yoga actually conserve and generate energy. (Vigorous exercise has its benefits, but for anyone coping with illness, conserving energy is a useful feature.)

- *Clearing the body of toxins.* The body is protected by the lymphatic system. You've probably noticed the swollen lymph glands in your neck when you have a sore throat. Lymph is a colorless fluid that washes through your system, carrying pollutants, internal toxins, and germs with it. In Qigong, for example, the rhythmic movements, deep breathing, and postures circulate the lymph, enhancing your immune function.

  Deepening the breath is the signal that stimulates the lymph system. The second factor that stimulates lymph circulation is movement — the act of contracting and releasing your muscles — but the movement does not need to be vigorous to have a beneficial effect on the system. One of the reasons gentle exercise is so spectacularly effective is that it efficiently activates the lymph system.

- *Delivering immune cells to their sites of activity.* The lymph is an important vehicle for the transport of both immune forces and artillery: T cells and certain antibodies.

- *Shifting out of the adrenaline mode.* Research has found that Qigong, for example, tends to promote the "relaxation response." This is a phase in which the body relaxes and rebuilds, shifting from adrenal hormone production during exertion or conflict to a rest-and-repair stage. In this mode, the body can produce the chemical messengers that call forth and activate immune cells. This shift is also important, because the presence of high levels of adrenal hormones in the human body can cancel out some of the activity of the immune cells.

- *Stimulation of the neurotransmitters that provide a sense of well-being.* The relaxation response is initiated through deep, slow breathing, coupled with relaxation.

The Importance of Oxygen

Research on the link between oxygen deficiency and disease has been active for several decades. Nobel Prize winner Otto Warburg found that oxygen deficiency was often associated with the development of cancer cells.[1] Studies that evaluated lung volume and oxygen capacity noted a parallel between reduced oxygen and disease, with reduced resistance to illness and increased mortality.[2,3] In studies of older subjects, immune deficiency was found to be one of the consequences of reduced oxygen metabolism.[4]

Oxygen plays a key role in our immune function. It is the source of the ammunition used by killer and natural killer T cells against viruses and tumors. Oxygen is converted into oxidants like peroxide and bleach (hypochlorite).[5] People who are ill or at risk for disease tend to exercise less, so there's less oxygen available to the body. By increasing the intake of oxygen and improving its circulation, therapeutic exercise such as Qigong and yoga can assist our immune function. Since this happens through gradual movement, focused breathing, and relaxation, these practices can be done by most anyone.

Typically, when we think of exercise, we think of aerobics, running, swimming, tennis — all vigorous activities intended to increase the supply of oxygen to the body (aerobic exercise means exercise "with oxygen"). We also exercise to build muscles, strengthen our heart, or to lose weight by burning up calories. Yet when those activities become more gradual and less intense, they still provide therapeutic benefits. In meditative exercise, since the metabolic resources promoted by the exercise are not expended as part of the physical activity, it is possible that it is more therapeutic. Done correctly, Qigong and yoga produce and circulate powerful internal resources for health and healing. In fact, aerobics, swimming, and walking can be modified to become more thera-peutic by slowing them down and focusing on the breath. At that point, Western exercise and ancient practice merge. Using this approach, walking can also take on a meditative form; in fact many religions include some type of walking meditation such as labyrinth walks or formal walking meditation. (See chapter 10 for more about exercise.)

According to the 1996 U.S. Surgeon General's Report on Exercise and Fitness, mild fitness practices are at least as beneficial as vigorous fitness practices. They may even be better, because there's also less risk of injury. Vigorous exercise reuses much of the energy that is created by the movement. Meditative practices such as yoga and Qigong conserve energy, and whenever healing is the goal, conserving energy is an important consideration.

Getting Started

Get a checkup. It's a good idea to get a checkup before you begin to exercise — especially if you have any special health condition or are over forty. Even then, the truth is that nobody is ever going to know as much about your strengths and limitations as you do. So when you exercise, be mindful and monitor yourself carefully. Any kind of pain is an important message from your body that some-thing may not right, like the red warning light on your dashboard. With all forms of exercise, it's important to pay attention to these messages and not to push yourself too far or too fast. Stay in the comfort zone.

Stay mindful. Some people approach exercising as if it's simply a function of the body and don't factor in the role of the mind. It's not uncommon to see people exercising on the StairMaster while reading the paper or riding an Exercyle while watching television. We encourage a different approach. Mindfulness can add a mean-ingful dimension to exercise. With relaxation and mindfulness, exercise accelerates the mind-body interaction. Increased awareness of your body and your health can support the healing process in different ways — it may provide insight that leads to more healthful behaviors or it may bring to mind important symptoms to share with your health-care practitioner. Mindfulness is an essential component of yoga, Qigong, and t'ai chi. The importance of mindfulness is now acknowledged throughout the world of sports — in major league football and basketball teams that use meditation; tennis and golf professionals who play practice the Zen of the game; and Olympic athletes who use visualization. Athletes describe this mindfulness as being "in the zone."

Take it easy. No matter what kind of exercise you've typically been doing or that you feel you should be doing, consider lessening the exertion a little and slowing the process down. Next, engage the breath meaningfully, in a deep, slow, relaxed, rhythmic fashion. Finally, adjust the mind toward a deep state of relaxation. By clearing the mind and refusing to engage in list-making and worrying, you curtail the adrenaline-based aspect of your nervous system activity. This activates a whole array of inner healing factors. Yoga, Qigong, and walking can be done anytime, anywhere. And each of these practices can be introduced very gradually, paced to your situation. None of these activities require equipment of any kind.

Qigong

Qigong (pronounced "chee-gung") is the umbrella of all the traditions of personal improvement and mind-body fitness from ancient Chinese culture. We know that these traditions probably predate the beginning of writing in China, around 500 B.C.E. Existing documents from that time indicate that the Chinese had already been using these practices for many hundreds of years.

The fact that Qigong and t'ai chi (a form of Qigong) have stood the test of time attests to their effectiveness. These fitness practices have been carefully refined for several thousand years. The various forms of practice can be categorized by their degree of activity, ranging from completely quiet to very dynamic. They include techniques that are performed in total stillness as meditation or meditative breathing exercises. Qigong and t'ai chi also involve gradual movement, like a dance in slow motion. Martial arts such as kung fu are vigorous forms of Qigong.

By most estimates, there are three to five thousand variations of Qigong. In all these forms, the primary focus is on the breath, to deepen and relax the breathing. At the same time, as an essential aspect of the practice, the mind is encouraged to relax in a state of meditation, clearing it of details or worries.

Benefits of Qigong

The medical literature includes hundreds of studies on the positive benefits of Qigong to promote health and overcome illness. Research on Qigong has shown positive results for patients with arthritis, asthma, cancer, chronic pain, diabetes, heart disease, high blood pressure, hepatitis, osteoporosis, stroke, and ulcers. Qigong was found to increase helper T cells by as much as 50 percent in a trainee group that had practiced Qigong for five months, compared to healthy volunteers who did not practice Qigong.[6] T'ai chi has been found to promote antibody production.[7]

Remember that if you have any type of health problem, before you begin to exercise, first seek guidance from a health-care practitioner. All the people in the research studies were under the supervision of a doctor.

- *A complement to treatment with medication,* Qigong was found to enhance improvement for patients being treated for asthma, high blood pressure, and cancer.[8]
- *Asthma.* Patients with asthma who practiced Qigong had reduced hospitalizations, took less sick leave, and needed fewer antibiotics.[9]
- *Chronic pain.* Of participants in this study who did Qigong, eighty-two reported less pain by the end of the first training session, and ninety-one had less pain by the last session weeks later.[10]

What to Do When You Can't Exercise

Lying-down Qigong can be very useful when we're sick, even if we spend a good deal of time just resting. We may think, "I can't exercise — I'm lying in bed." The Chinese would say, "No, you can exercise even when you're lying down. External movement is the least important part of this exercise. Internal activity is the essence of healing exercise practice."

Other Forms of Qigong

Initial Qigong practice, which is performed while completely still, can be accomplished lying down or sitting. To expand that practice, very gentle and small movements of hands, feet, and shoulders can be added. Next, as vitality improves, the practice can be done while sitting. Later, as more strength is developed, walking forms of Qigong can be added. T'ai chi is a beautiful form of walking Qigong. The most renowned form of this practice is called Guo Lin, named after a woman in China who had a very serious form of cancer and recovered using Qigong as a complement to her medical treatment. Guo Lin's form is one of the types of Qigong most frequently seen in the parks of China.

Other forms of walking Qigong include a series of graceful, philosophical movements associated with Taoism called the Wild Goose. Other dynamic forms are also described with poetic names: the Crane, Five Elements, Tendon Changing, Vitality, and Intelligence. Although some forms of Qigong are highly complex and difficult to learn, others are extremely simple. For example, t'ai chi involves 108 movements, which might take from six months to a year to learn. There are other types of Qigong that are very beneficial and yet can be learned in a few minutes. All forms of Qigong, from the simple to the most complex, offer the greatest improvement with regular practice over time.

Getting Started

If you find this practice appealing, seek out a class or private teacher. Simple Qigong exercises can be learned and practiced at home. Many hospitals and YMCAs have begun to offer Qigong or modified t'ai chi as a part of their mind-body programming. In a growing number of communities, it is possible to link up with a practice group either in a park or local recreation center. Some of these groups are offered without charge. In lieu of a class, a video can be helpful in learning some of the basic movements of Qigong but cannot totally replace a good teacher.

When Margaret was diagnosed with leukemia, she became more deeply involved with meditation and Qigong practice. Here's her experience in her own words:

An inner intuition seemed to direct me. I felt that anything I could do to increase my general health might also slow the progress of the disease.

Lab tests have shown that the leukemia has progressed slowly — slower than the doctor had expected. I feel my case is a great testimony to four things: the benefits of modern medicine, the prayers of my family, the vitamins and herbs that helped me to recover my energy after chemotherapy, and the gentle exercise and breathing practices I have done faithfully every day. Qigong and meditation are the rock on which I have built my healing and mental calm. Recently, I had a blood check, and my red and white cell counts had almost returned to normal. Two doctors have commented that they were surprised by these readings on someone who has been ill for so long. I take that as a very encouraging sign.

Yoga

Yoga is a subtle form of exercise that originated in India more than two thousand years ago. These ancient practices are recorded in the

200 B.C.E. Yoga Sutras of Patanjali in which the physical practice of hatha yoga is described as one of the Eight Limbs of Yoga. Hatha yoga can be complemented by other practices, which include breathing exercises, meditation, and karma yoga (acts of service).

The postures of this meditative exercise are designed to strengthen, stretch, and tone muscles and ligaments, with emphasis on particular regions of the body. In terms of modern fitness and training, yoga has come to mean the same thing as stretching. However, because it involves both the breath and the mind, yoga is much more than simple stretching. Its practices also encourage circulation while stimulating the secretions of glands and optimal function of the internal organs. In addition, the physical postures, breathing exercises, and meditation practices of yoga have been found to reduce stress, lower blood pressure, regulate heart rate, and even slow the aging process. Recent research has found benefit for a number of specific conditions, including asthma and heart disease.

In Ayurvedic medicine, hatha yoga is one of the lifestyle components a practitioner considers in developing an individual treatment program. Yoga has been documented to provide a subtle and powerful form of healing. It has also been adapted in Western forms of treatment such as the Ornish program. The programs developed by Dr. Dean Ornish address heart disease through a combination of medical management and lifestyle, including a yoga component.[11] And in the work of Jon Kabat-Zinn developed at the University of Massachusetts, research has documented the benefits of yoga in stress reduction and pain management, in settings that include offices, prisons, and hospitals.[12]

The essence of hatha yoga is the postures, or asanas, that poetically imitate the movements of animals and bear their names (the Cobra, the Lion, the Fish). Each posture is designed to stretch the muscles, flex the joints, and stimulate the internal organs and glands in various areas of the body. For example, the shoulder stand is thought to stimulate the thyroid gland through the gentle pressure of the chin on the throat area. The forward and the backward bend are designed to stretch and strengthen the muscles that surround the spinal column.

As the posture is performed, the body is gradually moved into position through a process of gentle stretching. The position is then held without moving, usually for less than a minute, while breathing slowly and deeply, and then the body is returned to a position of rest, lying outstretched or standing quietly. Yoga engages us in focused concentration, which adds a dynamic quality to the practice. A thorough session of yoga can provide the sense of deep relaxation experienced after a good massage.

Getting Started

Like Qigong, yoga requires no special equipment. All that is needed is a little space (an area about four by six feet) and a clean towel or pad on which to exercise. It can be done simply with the guidance of a good yoga book, as long as you are careful not to move too fast, stretch too far, or force your body. There are also helpful videos, and sometimes good yoga classes are shown on television. A live class can be more inspirational than a video or TV show, but it is important to work with a teacher who doesn't move too fast or too aggressively. Be wary of instructors who say things like "No gain without pain." The idea is to grow into the postures and become more flexible gradually, day-by-day. As helpful as videos and television are, yoga is about getting to know your own mind and body. Over time, you may find that your sessions move you into a deep state of inner focus and peacefulness.

Walking

We've been describing a more gradual approach to exercise. Almost any form of exercise can be modified to become more therapeutic. Vigorous aerobics can be adapted as low-impact aerobics, practiced with a dimension of mindfulness. Running becomes purposeful walking. With this approach, aerobic exercise, swimming, and walking can be modified to provide more of the therapeutic benefits gained from yoga or Qigong.

Why It's Worth Doing

Walking is one of the most overlooked forms of exercise. Many people think, "I walk all the time, what's so special about that?" You'll be encouraged to know that in the 1996 Surgeon General's report, walking was considered a preferred form of moderate exercise. Walking is also a perfect activity for most people who are not well enough to pursue more vigorous athletics and ideal for those who have health challenges but aren't drawn to forms of exercise like t'ai chi, Qigong, or yoga. Studies on the benefits of walking have found significant health improvement from a surprisingly brief investment of time.

- An hour of walking a week makes a difference.[13]
- Thirty minutes of walking a day is enough to promote fitness.
- Fifty minutes of walking, three times a week, increases T cell activity. Studies on the influence of moderate exercise training have shown that near-daily brisk walking (compared with inactivity) reduced the number of sickness days by half over a twelve- to fifteen-week period.[14]

No form of exercise will suit everyone. Even something as universal as walking may not be a match for you. For those readers who can't walk or who may be using a wheelchair, I would like to direct you to modified Qigong, yoga breathing, or other forms of gentle exercise that can be performed sitting.

Harry is an avid walker. His energy, sparkle, and pace suggest a man ten years younger. At seventy-five, Harry walks five miles every day, on his way to meetings and social events. He also thinks nothing of walking several miles to purchase fresh fish or to find bargains on regional produce. Highly active in public service and local politics, his calendar is filled with interesting and useful activities.

Getting Started

Walking benefits your circulation, delivering more oxygen to the body. In addition, deepening the breath, even while walking slowly, provides an acceleration of lymph circulation, which is a detoxification mechanism of the body. It is also possible to modify walking so that it is coupled with deep relaxation or meditation, which further activates the healing capacity of the nervous system.[15]

You can walk at a variety of paces. Purposeful walking is a little bit more like Qigong and yoga, and brisk walking is more like an aerobic activity. There's also race walking, which provides a strong cardiovascular stimulus. For anyone with health challenges, it is worth considering that slow, purposeful walking still provides the benefits of increased oxygen, more rapid circulation, and physical and mental stimulation yet generates very few oxidant by-products. In addition, the healing resources that are generated are not used up through exertion in the process. Here are some tips:

Begin slowly and build up. The 90-Day Fitness Program by Mark Fenton offers an excellent approach to getting started. Walk for five minutes on the first day and then add just a minute a day. If you do that, in ten days you'll be walking for fifteen minutes, and in a month you'll be walking more than a half an hour. By the end of the second month, if you wish, you could be walking an hour a day.

Build walking into your life. Another approach to walking is to build it into your life and your routine by making it part of the things you must do. As much as possible, group your errands in one location, park your car, and walk. When you're going to an appointment, if you can leave a little early, park a few blocks away (you may have to anyway!) and walk. Find other excuses to replace driving with walking. Remember to take the stairs at work or anywhere you happen to be.

Link walking to something you enjoy. If you like spontaneity, just remember to include a good walk in your activities each day. Although there's more aerobic benefit to be had from one long walk, several short brisk walks will still promote circulation. If the weather inspires you, take joyful walks on sunny days, romantic walks in the rain, or brisk walks in the wind. Bird watchers walk, shoppers walk, lovers walk.

Walk with a friend. Walking with someone else can be one of the best ways to walk and enjoy it. You may have a buddy with whom you walk regularly or friends with whom you go for long walks on the weekends or whenever you can. Enjoy!

Track your progress. If you value being organized, you will probably want to have a routine that's predictable, and you may find it satisfying to keep a log or a journal. If your doctor says you must walk, get a pedometer so you'll know how far you're actually walking, and you can celebrate your goals as you reach them.

My wife, Rebecca, and I have a favorite way of spending free time we call "just walking around." I may ask her on Thursday if she wants to plan something for Saturday, and she may say, "Why don't we just walk around?" That means no plan. It means we'll go for a walk and see where we end up. We could end up window-shopping, at the movies, hiking on the beach, or eating at a new restaurant or a favorite spot. So "just walking around" is a really fantastic combination of getting good (moderate) exercise, the fun of not knowing where you're going but knowing you will be with someone you like, or just out on your own on a surprise voyage of discovery.

✣

Roger Jahnke, O.M.D., is the author of the *The Healer Within,* now in its fourth printing, and *The Healing Promise of Qi.* A world expert on the practice of Qigong and chairman of the National Qigong Association, he lectures nationwide in venues that include Esalen, the Omega Institute, and the National Wellness Foundation. He also serves as a consultant to hospitals and health systems in the development of programs in health promotion and complementary and alternative medicine throughout the United States and overseas. His professional experience includes twenty years in the practice of traditional Chinese medicine and acupuncture. Roger Jahnke is director and CEO of Health Action in Santa Barbara, California. He can be reached at (805) 685-4670 or at (800) 824-4325. For more information on Qigong and t'ai chi, visit www.qigong-chikung.com.

Notes

1. O. Warburg, "The Prime Cause and Prevention of Cancer," Lindau Lecture, Wurzburg, Germany, K. Triltsch (1966).
2. T. Gordon and W. B. Kannel, *The Framingham Study: An Epidemiological Investigation of Cardiovascular Disease* (Bethesda, MD: National Heart and Lung Institute, 1970) sections 1–26.
3. K. Cullen et al., "Multiple Regression Analysis of Risk Factors for Cardiovascular Disease and Cancer Mortality in Busselton, West Australia: A 13-Year Study," *Journal of Chronic Diseases* 36 (1983): 371–377.
4. R. L. Saltzman et al., "Immunodeficiency of the Elderly," *Reviews of Infectious Diseases* 9, no. 6 (1987): 1127–1139.
5. J. Bland and S. H. Benum. *The 20-Day Rejuvenation Diet Program* (New York: NTC-McGraw Hill, 1999).
6. H. Ryu et al., "Effect of qigong training on proportions of T lymphocyte subsets in human peripheral blood," *American Journal of Chinese Medicine* 23, no. 1 (1995): 27–36.
7. Li, J. X., Y. Hong and K.M Chan, "Tai chi: physiological characteristics and beneficial effects on health," *British Journal of Sports Medicine* 35, no. 3 (2001): 148–156.

8. K. M. Sancier, "Therapeutic Benefits of Qigong Exercises in Combination with Drugs," *Journal of Alternative and Complementary Medicine* 5, no. 4 (1999): 383–389.

9. I. Reuther and D. Aldridge, "Qigong Yangsheng as a Complementary Therapy in the Management of Asthma," *Journal of Alternative and Complementary Medicine* 4, no. 2 (1998): 173–183.

10. W. H. Wu et. al., "Effects of Qigong on Late-Stage Complex Regional Pain Syndrome," *Alternative Therapies in Health and Medicine* 5, no. 1 (1999): 45–54.

11. D. Ornish, *Dr. Dean Ornish's Program for Reversing Heart Disease* (New York: Ballantine Books, 1990).

12. J. Kabat-Zinn, *Full Catastrophe Living: Using the Wisdom of Your Body and Mind to Face Stress, Pain, and Illness* (New York: Delta-Dell Books, 1990).

13. I. M. Lee et. al., "Physical activity and coronary heart disease in women: Is "no pain, no gain" passé?" *Journal of the American Medical Association* 285, no. 11 (2001): 1447–1454.

14. D. C. Meman and B. K. Pedersen, "Exercise and Immune Function: Recent Developments," *Sports Medicine* 27, no. 2 (1999): 73–80.

15. M. Fleshner, "Exercise and Neuroendocrine Regulation of Antibody Production: Protective Effect of Physical Activity on Stress-Induced Suppression of the Specific Antibody Response," *International Journal of Sports Medicine* 21, suppl. 1 (2000): S14–19.

CHAPTER SIX

Purification

Ellen Cutler, M.D., D.C.

Since toxicity is an inescapable part of life in the industrial world, we need to learn how to recognize and avoid toxins whenever possible and to cleanse ourselves from those we cannot avoid. For example, healing from food allergies means learning about the process of detoxification and making certain important changes in our lifestyle. Even small changes can go a long way toward helping to cleanse our system. In this chapter you'll find suggestions about simple methods of detoxification you can use at home to detoxify your body.

How Detoxification Supports Your Immunity

The immune system is a highly organized, powerful, system that protects your body from invasion by microorganisms. It also defends against cells (for example cancerous cells) that may develop incorrectly, which could cause harm to the body.

- *A system of barriers.* The immune system works by creating barriers to protect the cells from chemicals that could be toxic. It is also capable of recognizing foreign cells or microbes. The barriers are the skin and the mucosal membranes of the digestive tract, the genito-urinary system, and the respiratory system, which are vulnerable to toxins and microbes in food, water, or air.

- *A network of defenses.* This highly developed system can defend itself when these barriers are weakened and toxins enter the body. White cells attack and engulf toxins, providing vital protection. The immune system is not only tenacious but ferocious and comprehensive. Normally the immune system is strong enough to fight with every resource available. But toxicity, poor digestion, and allergies can play havoc with its performance. They reduce the efforts of our immune function by overloading, overburdening, and compromising its ability to defend the body, so detoxification is a primary and natural beginning to any healing process.

Immediate, practical approaches to detoxification include:

- Drinking enough water
- Juicing and fasting
- Breathing
- Dry skin brushing
- Detoxifying baths and saunas
- Cleansing the digestive tract
- Homeopathy
- Massage

Janet came to see me with severe chemical and environmental allergies. Like many people with these conditions, she had a high level of toxicity and poor detoxification. She was unable to live a normal life. She could not enter stores or even other people's homes unless she wore protection from environmental influences. Her sensitivities were essentially crippling her life. She could not work or take care of her family. She was devastated.

She came to my clinic pleading for help in overcoming this disability. My first approach with anyone is to gently and thoroughly detoxify the body through natural means, such as homeopathy, enzymes, and possible dietary changes including juicing and fasting. Although Janet was severely handicapped by these chemical and environmental allergies, she was surprisingly easy to work with. I recommended homeopathic remedies for kidney and colon detoxification and plant enzymes for adequate fat digestion and optimal digestive function. She was unable to tolerate fat in her diet, so her program included specific food allergy treatments she performed using home-allergy elimination treatment. I recommended that she return in two weeks for a reevaluation and another consultation.

Two weeks later, Janet returned with great news. Her symptoms were at least 70 percent better. Her environmental sensitivities were much less bothersome, and she was able to freely go many places she would not even have considered a few weeks ago. Her energy also returned. During the next few months she implemented deeper levels of detoxification, including exercise and periods of supervised fasting. She stated that she felt stronger, more able to fight infections for the first time in her life, and no longer disabled. She is now working and living a normal life.

How the Body Naturally Disposes of Toxins

When exposure to a toxin occurs, the body initially attempts to eliminate the toxic substance while still maintaining its full ability to function. We have many natural detoxification mechanisms. The organs that perform this task are the skin, lungs, gastrointestinal tract, kidneys, and liver.

We're bombarded every day with smog, dust, radiation, household chemicals, and pesticides. We also experience some degree of emotional stress at work and at home. In response our liver and our kidneys are continually conducting detoxification processes. This enables our cells to remain healthy and to produce the energy that sustains us.

Detoxification in the liver occurs in two phases. Phase One usually involves the transformation of toxic substances, in which chemicals, pesticides, or food additives are broken down through specific enzymes. As a result of this process, however, additional toxic and reactive by-products are created that need further detoxification — this is called Phase Two.

For example, the coal tar toxin in cigarette smoke is an inert substance until it is converted by Phase-One enzymes into a by-product — a metabolite that unfortunately happens to be highly toxic. This dangerous free radical can then cause severe tissue damage, or even cancer, if it is not further transformed. During Phase Two the body acts on these metabolites to further detoxify them, principally by increasing the body's ability to eliminate them through urine and bile. This process, which occurs moment by moment in our bodies, is of the utmost importance in preventing cellular damage and poor health.

If the level of toxicity is too great, before we know it, our physiology becomes overloaded. Important systems could be challenged and may be compromised. Then the digestive system may not function properly and the immune system can become overtaxed, unable to efficiently fight viruses and bacteria. This scenario also promotes premature aging, lack of sufficient energy, and poor enzyme production.

It begins to compromise the processes that ensure the healthy functioning of our cells. The result can be fatigue, depression, and possible allergic reactions to foods that we never reacted to before.

When the body is in a state of homeostasis, or balance, it has a strong capacity to accomplish detoxification efficiently. If you are struggling with food allergies, however, that could be an early warning sign that your system cannot adequately detoxify itself. In that case, intervention by a physician or well-trained health-care practitioner is needed. In fact, helping your body to detoxify is one of the first steps toward better immune function and optimal health.

How Do We Know When We Have Toxic Overload?

Any substance that is harmful or dangerous to the body and distorts our natural inner balance can be considered a toxin. When there is a condition of toxicity, the body will manifest physical imbalances. When the body's capacity to detoxify itself is exceeded, toxins are deposited both within and around the cells. This process causes a wide variety of health problems that are linked to many other more serious diseases, such as rheumatoid and osteoarthritis, multiple sclerosis, depression, and autoimmune diseases. The symptoms of toxicity may take years to manifest after an initial exposure to a toxin, making it difficult for one to discern the real source of the symptoms and the actual problem.

How do we know when we have a problem with toxicity? The truth is, physicians rarely see patients who do not have some kind of problem with toxins in their system. These substances are hard to avoid unless you are already aware of what causes toxicity and are actively doing some form of periodic cleansing.

Symptoms of toxicity commonly seen by health-care practitioners include symptoms that many readers will recognize in themselves:

- Headaches, mental confusion, or attention deficit disorder
- Exaggerated emotions, restlessness, or irritability

- Muscle pain, joint aches, or fatigue
- Nausea
- Dizziness
- Rashes, edema, or swollen glands

One of the values of detoxification is that it allows a clearer picture to emerge of what is actually occurring in the body. This was certainly the case with Harry, a man in midlife who had been ill for many years. His symptoms included severe burning and itching over his entire body, irritability, insomnia, dull nagging headaches, and nausea. He experienced one or more of these symptoms daily.

During his initial visit, Harry's responses to the extensive health-history questionnaire led me to conclude that he could be suffering from severe toxicity as well as allergies and could benefit from a detoxification regimen. Homeopathic remedies were prescribed that matched Harry's symptoms. When he returned two weeks later after a period of detoxification, all his symptoms had disappeared except for the headaches. I was then able to review his allergy tests to see if any allergies to foods might be the source of his headaches. After two months of BioSET Allergy Elimination Treatments, Harry no longer experienced headaches or any of his other symptoms and he was, in his own words, "as good as new."

Detoxification Methods

There are many different methods of detoxification that we can include in our daily lives. We live in our bodies twenty-four hours each day and often do not consider that, in the long run, eight hours of sleep a night is often not enough for them to adequately rest and regenerate. For this reason, it is important that we provide our bodies with additional opportunities for rest and cleansing, preferably several times a year.

Drinking Enough Water

Adequate water intake is essential for effective cleansing. One approach is to take a large sip of water every thirty minutes and to drink a whole glass an hour before eating your meals. I recommend using safe water not only for drinking but also for cooking, brushing your teeth, washing fresh food, and bathing and hand washing. (See chapter 4 for more information on the importance of water and how much we need daily.)

These days, acquiring safe water can be a problem because of the various possibilities of contamination. Even well water is no longer as safe as it once was because of contamination of the deeper water tables. I have also found that well water contains so many dissolved minerals that many sensitive people cannot tolerate it. Bottled water is definitely the recommended choice. Another way of removing unwanted contaminants from water is by filtering it. Although there are many types of filters on the market, most of them do not remove all undesirable elements from our drinking water, so if you decide to purchase a filter, do some research first. (See the resources at the end of the book for good sources of information and filter products.)

Juicing and Fasting

One activity that most of us can engage in regularly is periodic fasting. Fasting helps the body to heal and to resist diseases, infections, and toxins. It frees up the energy normally used for digestive functions so that this energy can be used elsewhere. Most important, fasting gives the body an opportunity to return to its natural state of homeostasis. During a fast, the body produces new healthy cells to replace old discarded ones and for cellular repair.

Many people make fasting a regular part of their lives, adopting a schedule of liquids only one day each week or liquids only for a three-day period once each month. Some even fast for as long as three to ten days at a time just on vegetable broth and vegetable juices.

Fasting when ill. When you are sick, it is important to let your body guide you regarding food intake. A rule of thumb is that if you can eat, you should. In other cases, appetite decreases and a natural fasting state occurs. This is due to temporary compromise of digestion as the metabolism speeds up and energy is directed away from the digestive tract. We can see this decreased capacity to digest in the tendency to have diarrhea or to vomit during illness. If the situation becomes severe, we may even require hospitalization and intravenous nutrition. This is usually not the time to embark on juicing and fasting: You do not want to deny your body the nutrients it may require to heal. At the same time, you don't want to overeat, since the digestive tract is often unable to handle large meals during illness. Again, let your body guide you.

When fasting may not be appropriate. For people who are not well nourished in general, juicing and fasting may be inappropriate without medical supervision. People who are thin or who don't receive optimum nutrition may not get the critical nutrients they need. They may become magnesium or potassium deficient, which can cause cardiac rhythm disturbances that could be fatal. Fasting in this case should be done under the supervision of a qualified health-care practitioner.

Maximum Nutrition

To get the most out of your fruit and vegetable drinks, it is often best to do the juicing yourself rather than buying the drinks commercially. To ensure that your juices are pure and full of nutrients, you should use organically grown produce as often possible so that harmful pesticides and chemical residues don't end up in your juice. If you are unable to obtain organically grown fruits and vegetables, make sure you peel or thoroughly wash your produce, using a vegetable brush to remove chemical residues and waxes. Most health food stores carry vegetable washes that help remove residues.

Fresh vegetable juices boost the immune system, remove toxins, and help the body to achieve homeostasis. The juices I have used most often over the years are beet, carrot, cabbage, celery, cucumber, kale, parsley, turnip, spinach, and watercress. I do not recommend using carrot juice on its own, since carrots are higher in natural sugars than other vegetables. Since most individuals are sensitive to sweeteners and sugar — even those found in nature — they can compromise homeostasis and effective detoxification. However, carrot juice is excellent for sweetening other juices when used in moderation. Strongly flavored vegetables, such as broccoli, celery, onions, parsley, rutabaga, and turnips should also be used in small amounts.

Green Drinks

Green drinks, which use a lot of green, leafy vegetables, raw sprouts, and grasses as their primary ingredient also cleanse the body of pollutants and have a rejuvenating effect. The chlorophyll in these drinks helps to purify the blood and detoxify the body. Green juices can be made using alfalfa sprouts, celery, dandelion greens, spinach, cabbage, and wheat grass. I sometimes sweeten my green drinks with fresh carrot or apple juice. Green juices have great health benefits, but they are very potent. People who have digestive problems or other chronic disorders may want begin with no more than eight to ten ounces a day.

A good recipe for a green drink is:

1 beet, including tops
1 large handful of spinach
1 large handful of kale
4 to 5 carrots

Blend

During fasting, you should make sure you drink at least eight glasses of liquid each day. It is also a wise idea to use distilled water to dilute juices from fresh fruits and vegetables to prevent your digestive process from being overloaded. It is good to take vitamin and mineral supplements when eating normally, but do not take them while fasting because they can interfere with the cleansing process. (Note: I only recommend distilled water during fasts. Otherwise, use bottled spring water because it contains the natural minerals.)

Warm Vegetable Broth

If you prefer a hot drink during fasting, vegetable broths are recommended. Here is the recipe for my favorite broth:

- 3 stalks celery
- 2 red potatoes, unpeeled
- 3 medium beets with tops
- 4 carrots
- 1 onion
- 1 clove garlic

Cover and simmer for 45 minutes. Remove the vegetables, and blend up the broth and drink it when it has cooled down.

Once you are ready to break your fast, gradually return to solid foods over the course of three to four days. Start out by eating lightly, and always chew your foods well. This enhances the digestive process.

A fast that lasts longer than three days should not be undertaken without medical supervision.

Breathing

Breathing, one of the only functions of the body that we can perform both consciously and unconsciously, is an important and very basic cleansing method. It can help cleanse the body both physically and mentally. Breathing is also directly connected to our emotional states, all of which affect the speed, depth, and regularity at which we breathe. For example, anger, which makes us take quick, shallow breaths, can be calmed by breathing slowly, deeply, quietly, and regularly. Most people do not realize that stressful emotions can limit the body's ability to detoxify. For this reason, learning some appropriate breathing techniques can be profoundly cleansing.

One detoxifying breathing technique, described in *Radical Healing* by Rudolph Ballentine, M.D., is diaphragmatic breathing. To do this exercise, lie on you stomach on a firm surface such as the floor with your forehead resting comfortably on your crossed arms, or lie on your back with a three-pound object, such as a large Ziploc-type bag filled with sand, on your belly. The goal of this exercise is to practice effortless breathing in the midriff rather than in the belly or chest. This is achieved by simply holding in your abdominal muscles as you inhale so that the lower edges of your rib cage are pushed outward, expanding the diaphragm. This breathing exercise promotes calmness and quietness and releases blocked energy pathways, promoting cleansing and revitalization. It also targets emotional cleansing, helping to release tension.

The delivery of oxygen and removal of carbon dioxide determines the efficiency of functioning for all body systems. The body cannot cleanse itself, heal itself, or maintain life without the oxygen supplied by breathing. The motions of respiration mechanically pump lymphatic fluid throughout the system and assist circulation. If breathing is restricted, fluid collects, causing edema and the buildup of waste products from cellular metabolism. If we could all just remember to take in a deep breath and release it slowly, periodically throughout our stressful, chaotic, activity-filled days, we would derive great detoxifying benefits.

Dry Skin Brushing

Dry skin brushing is an important tool for skin cleansing and detoxification. This technique involves briskly brushing the entire body with a dry vegetable or soft bristle brush before showering or bathing in the morning or evening. Begin with the soles of your feet and work up to the top of your legs in large broad strokes. When you get to the top part of your body, brush from the palms of the hands toward the shoulders. Always aim in the direction of the lymph nodes located in the groin and underarm areas. Never brush the nipples or the face, and always brush toward the heart when doing the chest and back area. I recommend brushing for about five minutes three times a week. This is far superior for skin cleansing to any bath or shower.

Detoxifying Baths and Saunas

Detoxification baths help eliminate toxins by activating fluid movement in the tissues and increasing perspiration. Several substances may be used in the bath to aid in detoxification.

Epsom salts. I have always favored Epsom salts because they promote relaxation and calmness. These salts work as a counterirritant on the skin to increase blood supply. The sulfur content of Epsom salts also aids in detoxification. You should begin with $\frac{1}{4}$ cup of Epsom salts and gradually increase the amount with each bath until you are using four cups per tub of clean water.

Herbal and clay baths. These products are available in a variety of forms. Although clay is most frequently used in compresses or packs, the drawing action of clay in the bath also aids in detoxification. Use $\frac{1}{2}$ cup of clay to a tub of water. There are several types of clay on the market, and all are appropriate for bathing. The clay sold specifically for bathing will not clog up your drain.

Saunas. This technique also provides detoxification. Since it is difficult for the body to mobilize toxins out of fatty tissue (where most of them are stored), it is important to find ways to aid the body in clearing these toxins. A sauna is a relatively airtight room with wooden platforms and benches. The air is kept fresh by a special ventilation system that preheats outside air before it enters the sauna. There are two basic types of saunas, dry and moist, and both are kept at a temperature of about 140 to 150 degrees Fahrenheit. This can be a very effective tool for releasing stored toxins from the cells.

When looking for a sauna to use in your detoxification program, seek a dry sauna that has been constructed to be environmentally safe, with air cleaners attached to the air circulation units. Although most commercial saunas found in health clubs are safe, some tend to be too hot, have inadequate levels of oxygen, and are not environmentally well constructed. For this reason, become knowledgeable about saunas. I recommend dry saunas because they increase sweating and speed detoxification. Be sure to replace the fluids you have lost due to perspiration. Drink plenty of water, both while you are in the sauna and afterward to keep your kidneys flushing out the toxins. Then allow yourself a period of rest. The body needs a quiet time to adjust and rebalance itself.

Cleansing the Digestive Tract

Detoxification would not be complete without considering the organs of elimination. Our primary detoxification organs are the liver and the colon. During times of stress and acute overload, cleansing these organs will help to restore their optimal function.

Liver health. The liver is a major organ for the processing and elimination of toxic wastes. It breaks down all the chemicals we are exposed to every day, such as pollution, drugs, or cleaning agents. The liver also metabolizes hormones such as estrogen that are used in regulating the body's processes. If the liver is unable to process estrogen adequately owing to a toxic overload, excess estrogen results. This can lead to high blood pressure and breast, uterine, and vaginal cancer. The liver also metabolizes testosterone. Elevated levels of this hormone can cause aggressiveness and mood swings as well as excess sexual energy. Because the liver also filters the blood, an overburdened liver will not be able to adequately eliminate toxins from the blood. These unfiltered toxins can then infiltrate the liver cells, potentially causing irreversible damage.

A poorly functioning liver can cause poor digestion, gas, constipation, soreness in the liver area, skin problems such as acne or psoriasis, mood swings, or emotional excesses. Unmetabolized toxins that can result are circulated throughout the body, which can lead to disease. If you have several of these symptoms, you might consider a liver cleansing to help stimulate the elimination of toxic wastes from the body. I use a liver enzyme made from an herbal enzyme formula (WellZyme Liver) that helps to increase liver detoxification as well as restoration of its function (see the Resources at the back of the book). Another product I have used in my practice for many years is UltraClear by Metagenics. This powder can be used to replace or supplement a meal and supplies antioxidants and amino acids that support liver cleansing and revitalization. Other factors that can stimulate liver detoxification are minimizing protein intake; using only small amounts of unsaturated fats; eating foods such as garlic, onions, and broccoli; reducing refined sugar; and eating green, moderately bitter vegetables such as endive, collards, dock, and dandelion.

One of the best liver cleansers that I have found is coffee enemas, which is useful in ridding the body of toxins and accumulated waste products. This is a low-volume enema that mainly stays in the end of the colon, the area where the colon and the liver are connected through the circulatory system. Toxins in this part of the colon are sent to the liver for detoxification rather than being circulated throughout the body. Therefore, a coffee enema can speed up the emptying of the bowel, increasing liver detoxification. The caffeine has the added advantage of not washing out minerals and electrolytes. Individuals who are very sensitive to caffeine are usually not affected, because the caffeine goes primarily into the colon-liver circulation area, not into the entire system. Warning: People with gallstones should not take coffee enemas.

Digestive health. A healthy colon is of utmost importance in detoxification. A colon that is toxic or not performing optimally causes backup and fermentation of fecal material. When this happens, bacterial infections or parasitic infestations can develop, which make the system toxic. These infestations can also adversely affect the emotions and cause many other symptoms, from migraines to sciatica to psychological disorders. Eventually, the very integrity of our cells will be affected, limiting their ability to produce energy and fight disease.

Ultimately, good digestion is the key to good colon health. Take measures to chew and digest your food sufficiently, eat a balanced diet that is suited to your needs, and drink enough water to keep your colon healthy. Good digestive health is the basis for the vitality of the rest of the body.

Homeopathy

Some of the most effective tools for detoxification that I use in my own practice are homeopathic formulas. Used alone or along with the detoxification methods described above, homeopathy can help you to achieve detoxification quickly and effectively.

Homeopathy is a medical system developed two hundred years ago by a German physician, Dr. Samuel Hahnemann. The system is based on the philosophy, "Let likes be cured with likes." Dr. Hahnemann believed that the body's responses to illness are an effort to heal itself and discovered that giving a person a remedy that causes those same symptoms can actually help give the healing process a boost. Based on this idea, Hahnemann developed the system of homeopathy, using minute doses of specific substances as homeopathic remedies. He also believed that what was really being treated was a person's "vital force," the body's fundamental energy and vitality. A well-chosen remedy is intended to activate the vital force to promote greater healing. The change in vital force determines the success of the homeopathic remedy given to the patient. When Hahnemann experimented with different potencies of his remedies, he found that the more diluted substances had even fewer side effects and acted longer and more deeply on the body and thus were more effective.

Over the years, working with thousands of patients to identify and eliminate their food allergies, I have gotten the best and most long-lasting results in allergy clearing when clients also detoxify, using homeopathic remedies. These remedies are most effective when used in the beginning stages of healing. They usually work quickly and deeply, cause very few side effects, and are not allergenic. While they gently and effectively cleanse the system, they also treat the body's vital force and energy. Patients and practitioners report that when a well-chosen homeopathic remedy is taken, symptoms begin to decrease almost immediately.

Homeopathic detoxification preparations stimulate the cells to release toxic residue. Once this process occurs, the body will begin to filter out this residue through the organs of elimination. Sometimes, depending on their toxic load, a person can experience adverse reactions such as an increased need for sleep, anxiety, nervousness, bad breath, frequent urination, or softer stools. After the elimination process is complete, most people feel an increase in energy, a heightened sense of well-being, and a greater resistance to colds and flu. Begin slowly. If increasing the dosage causes uncomfortable reactions, cut back. There is no rush. These remedies will work even if you use only two drops as opposed to five or six. The process might just take slightly longer.

While taking homeopathic remedies, remember to drink water, exercise, and breathe. Practice good eating habits. Chew your food well so that the enzymes in your mouth can enhance the digestive process; eat simply; reduce your intake of refined sugar, junk food, excess salt, and other processed foods. Avoid foods to which you know you have an intolerance.

Joselyn, a twenty-eight-year-old teacher, was so plagued by chronic fatigue that she was barely able to maintain her teaching schedule. Shortly after starting treatment, she faxed a letter to my office. It said, "Dear Doctor, I've been on your homeopathic remedy for nine days now and I have more energy today than I've had in two years. I am encouraged."

Massage

Massage is another excellent complement to any detoxification program. Our bodies respond both externally and internally to friction on the skin, pressure on deeper tissues, and sensory input around the joints. Our bodies rely on the movement of fluids to function well, and massage is an effective means of promoting fluid circulation. To survive and function, every cell must continuously receive nutrients, water, and oxygen — while expelling toxic wastes. This cycle requires good circulation. Massage increases circulation, which facilitates cleansing and the removal of waste materials from the lymph system throughout the body. In brief, the cleansing action of massage promotes elimination of toxins, improves blood and lymph circulation, increases oxygen supply to cells, and eliminates excess fluid in the muscles and tissues.

Any type of massage also directly affects the nerves, organs, and circulation and indirectly affects the body as a whole. Massage can help the body and mind cope with stress and pain. We all know the ability of soothing, comforting touch to moderate shock, distress, or fear. There is actually a physiological basis for this effect. The nerve pathways carrying the sensation of touch to the brain are thicker, faster, and more numerous than the pathways that carry pain messages. By distracting the body from pain through touch, it is able to receive impulses to relax. As relaxation continues, contracted muscles are also released. When pain is lessened, a person is better able to evaluate a stressful situation.

All massage techniques work by stimulating specific receptors in the skin, resulting in a particular response, depending on the type of massage used. Let me caution you that some physical conditions preclude vigorous, stimulating, or deep massage. Before requesting bodywork, take under consideration your physical condition and any extraordinary circumstances. Note that massage therapy is contraindicated for those with advanced heart disease, kidney failure, phlebitis, tumors, or conditions associated with bleeding or bruising. Clearly people with skin infections, wounds, new scar tissue, or burns would also be inappropriate candidates for massage unless it is provided under the direction of a doctor or physical therapist.

Basic types of massage include soft-tissue massage, connective tissue and fascia massage, massage of the meridians, and energy work and healing touch.

Swedish massage is the most familiar style of soft-tissue bodywork. It involves treatment of the entire external body, except for the reproductive organs. A person receiving this type of massage is always draped and may undress to the degree that is personally comfortable. Oil, powder, or alcohol are the mediums most often used to help the therapist's hands glide smoothly over the skin surface. Swedish massage stretches the limbs and actively stimulates the skin and soft tissue.

Manual lymphatic massage is a specific technique that requires training and should only be practiced by a massage professional. In this type of massage, the skin is kneaded but never stroked. The effect of lymphatic massage is largely mechanical, displacing fluids and the substances that the lymph carries, so the techniques must be executed precisely. The more exact the technique, the more effective the results.

Connective tissue/fascia massage involves massaging the fascia, the part of our bodies that fastens the muscles to the bones and the bones to the joints. The fascia surrounds every nerve and vessel, holds all internal structures in place, and envelops the body as a whole. This type of massage is applied through direct pressure, squeezing, kneading, and stretching muscle tissue and limbs. The goal is to move large amounts of toxins and wastes out of the intercellular fluids and into the bloodstream, where they can be eliminated.

Rolfing, another method of deep massage, uses fingers, knuckles, forearms, elbows, and sometimes even special tools to stretch or exert pressure on the body's connective tissues in an effort to energize and reshape them. This pressure and stretching, carefully applied at specific points and in specific directions, softens and lengthens the connective tissues to make them more malleable. This promotes detoxification and cleansing of the system. Rolfing also improves the structural properties of the connective tissue.

Shiatsu massage, a form of acupressure developed in Japan, has been described as a dance along the meridians of the body. The practitioner uses body weight, rather than muscle strength, to apply pressure on the meridians with hands or fingers. The pressure is applied rhythmically, up and down various meridians. The practitioner uses the balls of the fingers, the thumbs, and the base of the thumb in a combination of eleven specific positions. This technique can help to reduce muscle tension by stimulating the point along the meridian that is related to the particular muscle or joint. This technique is effective for overall cleansing of the body as well as for specific ailments such as migraines, stiff neck, and sciatica.

Reflexology is a method of foot massage that originated in China. It is referred to as a "zone therapy," because the specific pressure points stimulated on the feet reflect the entire body — each foot represents one half of the body. Treatment consists of using the thumbs to apply firm pressure. Working on these reflexes can cleanse the body, relieve headaches, clear congested sinuses, reduce the pain of menstrual cramps, ease backaches, and reduce swelling.

Our efforts to enhance immune function are most effective when they include avenues to detoxify, restore digestion, and eliminate allergies. This must be emphasized in regaining and maintaining total health and maximum longevity.

❧

Ellen Cutler, M.D., D.C., holds a medical degree from University of California, Los Angeles; a degree in chiropractic from Western States Chiropractic College in Portland, Oregon; and extensive postgraduate training that includes women's health, nutrition, and enzyme therapy. Dr. Cutler is author of three books: *Winning the War against Asthma and Allergies, Winning the War against Immune Disorders and Allergies,* and most recently, *The Food Allergy Cure.* Dr. Cutler is developer of the BioSET method, a form of applied acupressure that has been found highly effective in the treatment of food allergies and is now used worldwide. Further information on BioSET for the public and for health-care professionals is available by calling the BioSET Institute at (877) 927-0741 or visiting their website at www.bioset-institute.com.

food:friend
or foe

Digestion — The Best-Kept Secret

Len Saputo, M.D.

Eating Your Way to Health

Jerry Stine, N.C.

Allergies and Sensitivities

Michael Rosenbaum, M.D.

CHAPTER SEVEN

Digestion — The Best-Kept Secret

Len Saputo, M.D.

One of the best-kept secrets is that the digestive tract is the largest immune organ in the body. Surprisingly, the majority of our body's immune defenses reside there. They are strategically located for our protection, because this is the site of entry for potentially dangerous microbes and chemicals that enter our bodies with food and water. When this large and strategically placed immune system isn't working well, our defenses are lowered. Once our barriers are down, it may not be possible to keep the ecology of the intestinal tract in balance. And it becomes more difficult to defend ourselves against invaders.

Immunity and Digestion

The vitality of our immune system is maintained through an inner system of checks and balances.[1] Two primary components of our immunity in the digestive tract are the friendly flora and our antibodies. The third major factor is the efficiency of our digestion.

- *The friendly flora crowd out potentially harmful bacteria, just as healthy grass crowds out weeds.* In this way, they prevent the overgrowth of yeast such as candida or harmful bacteria such as *Clostridium difficile.*[2] The beneficial bacteria also manufacture certain essential nutrients.

- *Efficient digestion can also minimize the overgrowth of yeast and bacteria.* If food is incompletely digested, it can create an environment that is hospitable to certain yeast or bacteria. This can cause imbalance in the ecology of the digestive tract and create another burden on immunity.[3]

- *Through digestion is also important in minimizing allergies that can drain our immunity.* Our immune artillery actually attacks large undigested food molecules as if they were the "enemy." So poorly digested food can add yet another burden to the immune system.[4,5] Essentially, supporting optimal digestion preserves our immune capacity.

Before Carol entered college, she was hardly sick a day in her life. That first semester at Berkeley was really tough. She stayed up late studying, gulped down fast food, and when she wasn't at the library, she was socializing. Cold season hit just before finals, and Carol was one of the first to catch a cold — a cold that wouldn't go away. She saw her doctor, who prescribed several courses of antibiotics, because she felt she couldn't afford to be sick. Unfortunately, it took about three months before the cold went away.

But Carol was never the same again. She began to have recurring yeast infections and bouts of colitis. Her yeast infections were brought under control with medication — in addition, the digestive problems required treatment with muscle relaxants and tranquilizers. Even then she almost never felt well. She was finally told to see a psychiatrist, who suggested that her digestive problems were probably related to her nerves. When Carol came to see me, she had suffered from this condition for more than ten years. By that time, she'd had every test in the book, including X rays, blood work, and even a colonoscopy, but all the lab texts came back with normal results.

Carol was beginning to believe that she really was losing her grip on reality. I requested lab tests (the comprehensive digestive stool analysis or the C.D.S.A.) to analyze her digestive capacity and found she had a major imbalance of intestinal microflora — a severe overgrowth of yeast and a deficiency of normal beneficial bacteria. We devised a nutritional program to support healing of the digestive tract — a diet low in sugar, with anti-yeast herbs, antioxidant nutrients, and generous supplementation of friendly bacteria. Within ten days, Carol's symptoms cleared, and she has remained free of this condition ever since. About every four to six months, we have lab work done to check her flora levels. For the past two years, she has slowly redeveloped healthy microflora. Carol has discontinued psychotherapy and is beginning to feel like her old self.

Inner Balance

Nature's incredible perfection is exemplified par excellence in the complex ecological balance that exists between the microflora in the digestive tract and its human host. When the host and the microflora coexist in harmony, a healthy state of symbiosis results. In a sense this is extraordinary, since more than five hundred different species of bacteria reside in the digestive tract and collectively produce more metabolic activity than any other organ system in our body.[6,7,8] As a result, our digestive flora have been equated to an entire organ or system within itself. When symbiosis is disrupted, this disordered state is described as dys-symbiosis, or "dysbiosis." Such a disordered ecology often disturbs our inner balance and can ultimately result in disease.[9,10]

We hardly ever think about the flora in our bodies, and their importance is usually underestimated. But research shows that even with conditions as serious as AIDS and cancer, good flora can enhance health and perhaps even prolong life. The loss of balance in the digestive flora — dysbiosis — occurs far more often than we usually appreciate. Basically, any situation that can alter the physical integrity or the biochemical balance of the gastrointestinal (GI) tract can result in changes in the microflora. This destroys some of the beneficial flora and can allow harmful microbes to take over or "overgrow."

Normally the immune system keeps the bacteria in check, so abnormal dysbiosis may not progress to a disease state. When dysbiosis does occur, it signals a loss of homeostasis that requires attention. Even when inner balance is lost, the disturbed ecology may not result in immediate symptoms. Rather, this type of condition often underlies a vague sense of unwellness or mild symptoms such as fatigue, malaise, or poor digestion — but nothing that adds up to a specific diagnosis or an identifiable disease. The loss of inner balance may occur gradually.

Resistance to infection or overgrowth depends on the individual's level of stress and the quality of diet, habits, and lifestyle. Those who already have impaired immunity are likely to be more vulnerable. Imbalances can be caused by almost any factors that compromise digestion or immunity, such as poor diet, chronic stress, infection or inflammation, use of antibiotics, or exposure to toxins. Secondary conditions can develop due to dysbiosis, ranging from allergies to arthritis or asthma. See the following table for causal and resulting conditions associated with flora imbalances.

Flora Imbalance

Major Causes to Flora Imbalance	Conditions Linked to Flora Imbalance
• Poor diet	• Arthritis (both chronic and rheumatoid)
• Stress	• Attention deficit disorder
• Antibiotic or drug therapy	• Autistic-like symptoms
• Decreased immune status	• Chemical sensitivities
• Inflammation	• Chronic fatigue syndrome
• Decreased gut motility	• Food allergies and intolerances
• Poor digestion	• Inflammatory bowel disease
• Intestinal infection	• Irritable bowel syndrome
• Presence of toxins	• Joint conditions
• Increased intestinal acidity	• Compromised liver function
	• Malnutrition
	• Symptoms that resemble schizophrenia
	• Skin disorders (such as acne, dermatitis, and eczema)

Adapted with permission from the monograph *Comprehensive Digestive Stool Analysis Application Guide,* Great Smokies Diagnostic Laboratory, Asheville, North Carolina; © 1998.

The Role of Immunity in Preventing Dysbiosis

By themselves harmful microflora are rarely the single cause of dysbiosis. The essential questions to ask are: What is happening that enables some of these organisms to overgrow and upset the balanced ecology that previously existed? It's important to remember that most of the microbes that cause illness are normally present in small numbers — for example, staph are almost always found in the body, and strep are present an estimated 40 percent of the time

What makes an organism that is normally benign become harmful or pathogenic? Microbes that cause an overgrowth often indicate that immune defenses have been compromised. Again, we know this because most microbes that overgrow in the digestive tract are not in themselves harmful until they have the opportunity to predominate over the beneficial bacteria. Two primary factors determine just how extensive and destructive an overgrowth will become — the strength of the microbe and the strength of our resistance.

The first factor is the capacity of the microbe to overgrow and produce toxins that can injure us — this determines its "virulence." The second is the vitality of our immune defenses. We tend to overlook this factor, unless the underlying disease is severe, as in AIDS, for example. It is widely believed that invading organisms are the primary cause of illness and that destroying them is the solution. But most of the organisms that normally inhabit the intestinal tract can cause serious illness under certain conditions.[11] For example, various yeast such as candida are present in almost everyone. Women in particular find that stress or illness can leave them vulnerable to an overgrowth of the resident candida. In people with AIDS, this same harmless yeast may viciously attack the body because of the absence of immune defenses.

When we think of harmful microbes, we think of dramatic examples of bacteria such as toxic *E. coli* or salmonella. However, posing an equal or sometimes even greater risk are the subtle changes that can occur in the digestive tract. They don't result from these "killer bacteria" but from the gradual shift in the ecology of the digestive tract. As the body shifts from perfect harmony and interdependence — symbiosis — to a state of disharmony or dysbiosis, there is a subtle and accumulative adverse effect on the state of our health. This is the fundamental nature of dysbiosis.

Once the inner ecology shifts, at some point symptoms begin to manifest. But the ecology may be disturbed long before a specific illness becomes apparent and can be diagnosed. The point at which identifiable symptoms occur will depend on the strength of the microbe and the strength of immune defenses. Once an overgrowth occurs, a gradual loss of optimal health can result. As the body is weakened, additional harmful microbes come into play through a gradual process in which the dysbiosis deepens and becomes more severe. At that point, the body becomes vulnerable to a number of conditions. In some cases, resident bacteria may overgrow in such numbers that they become harmful, and the volume of their toxic output then begins to affect the body. In other situations, the body becomes more vulnerable to invasion from microbes coming in with food or water. Salmonella or giardia are good examples. Once there are significant levels of these pathogenic microbes in the body, eventually symptoms of infection will develop.

Causes of Imbalance

A number of basic lifestyle factors can set the stage for loss of balance in digestive ecology.

Diet. It should not be a surprise that what we eat can affect which organisms will have a growth advantage in the digestive tract. Each bacterial species has specific nutritional needs that, if met, will allow it to enjoy accelerated growth. The normal, friendly bacteria that inhabit the gut survive best on high-fiber diets.[12] If we consume adequate amounts of fiber, these bacteria will have the nutrition and the growth advantage they need to flourish. Certain types of overgrowth are associated with a diet high in starches and sugars — resulting in a type of dysbiosis linked to "excess fermentation." This bacterial overgrowth may also worsen digestion.[13] (See chapter 8 for additional information on achieving balance in the diet.) Diets high in fat and meat and low in fiber lead to what is termed "putrefactive dysbiosis."[14]

In this situation, a harmful bacteria called bacteroides tends to proliferate and results in the overproduction of ammonia. In addition, the body's production of certain essential nutrients decreases and can lead to nutritional shortages throughout the digestive tract. This type of dysbiosis is also associated with elevated levels of bile acids, which increase the risk for colon cancer, and elevated estrogen levels, which are linked to an increased risk for breast cancer.[15]

Digestion. Failure to digest food typically occurs because of low stomach acid or digestive enzymes (see the following table). Incompletely digested food and nutrients are then able to reach the lower small intestine and colon. This poorly digested food can have an adverse effect, because it provides fuel to support overgrowth of many potentially harmful bacteria.[16,17]

Not Enough Enzymes	
Symptoms of Low Enzyme Levels	**Disorders Linked to Low Enzymes**

• Decreasing levels that parallel aging	• Allergies and sensitivities
	  - Wheat or gluten intolerance
	  - Lactose and dairy intolerance

• Poor absorption of nutrients	• Lactose and dairy intolerance

• Deficiency in some specific nutrients, but not others (difficult to identify)	• Inflammatory disorders
	  - Crohn's disease
	  - Gastroenteritis

• Evidence of undigested fats in lab results	• Parasitic disorders
	  - Giardia infection
	  - Cryptosporidium infection

• Deficiency of essential fatty acids	
• Low energy due to lowered calories	

Adapted with permission from the monograph *Comprehensive Digestive Stool Analysis Application Guide,* Great Smokies Diagnostic Laboratory, Asheville, North Carolina; © 1998.

Overuse of antibiotics may be the most frequent cause of significant dysbiosis. When antibiotics are used, profound changes occur in the consistency of the microflora in the GI tract and throughout the body. If host defenses are adequate, and the ecological balance is not too deeply disturbed, the normal microflora may be able to reestablish their beneficial symbiotic relationship. However, when there is repeated or prolonged antibiotic treatment, especially in the presence of inadequate immune defenses, a state of severe and sustained dysbiosis may develop, which can result in disease. In this situation, the microflora are substantially reduced, and the resulting condition is termed "deficiency dysbiosis."[18] Again, another factor in deficiency dysbiosis is the inadequate consumption of fiber, the major source of nutrition for normal flora.

One of the most dreaded iatrogenic diseases that too often develops in this situation is infection by the bacteria *Clostridium difficile,* a potentially life-threatening complication of antibiotic usage. It is ironic that conventional medical treatment of this condition is almost always to use additional antibiotic therapy aimed at stopping the clostridium overgrowth. While this approach may be successful at times, it reflects the too-common perspective of "us against the germs." This approach focuses on killing the microbes that are invading the body or taking over the digestive tract, without focusing on the underlying process affecting microflora ecology.

Inflammatory conditions of the intestinal tract include Crohn's disease, ulcerative colitis, and infection by a variety of agents (bacterial, viral, fungal, or parasitic microorganisms). Inflammation can disrupt and damage the intestinal lining and cause the loss of normal defenses that prevent the growth of bacteria. Then a wide variety of opportunistic organisms can take advantage of this change in environment and create an ecological shift of the microflora. Many of the by-products of this new microflora are toxic to the digestive tract and cause further damage to the tissue, creating a self-perpetuating, vicious cycle.

Exposures to environmental toxins are increasing at an alarming rate. Many toxic substances find their way into the digestive tract on food with pesticide residues or additives. Our water also contains contaminants such as chlorine and fluoride. In addition, our drinking water can accidentally become contaminated by industrial chemicals, petroleum products, heavy metals, or other toxins. We also ingest small amounts of toxins from products such as toothpaste, mouthwashes, and numerous other sources, including our dental fillings. These substances can cause damage to the lining of the intestinal tract and to the beneficial microflora. Toxins can also cause changes in our inner balance, lower our resistance, and set the stage for the development of dysbiosis. A wide variety of products can have profound effects on the balance of the gut microflora, including pharmaceutical drugs such as antacids; drugs that block acid production; anti-inflammatory drugs (NSAIDs) such as ibuprofen; birth control pills; steroids; some chemotherapy treatments; and various other medications.[19] (See chapter 11 for additional information about minimizing exposure to allergens and toxins.)

Stress can have profound effects on the digestive tract. Many people develop digestive symptoms when they're in high-stress situations, because stress can lower defenses in the digestive tract.[20,21] In addition, the completeness of the digestive process is related to the time it takes food to pass through the intestinal tract (transit time), and this process can also be altered by the effects of stress. (See chapters 12 and 13 for more information about minimizing the effects of stress, both mentally and physically.)

Effects on Immunity

If the beneficial flora in the digestive tract declines because of heavy antibiotic use or a poor diet, harmful flora can overgrow. As we've discussed, these flora primarily include yeast and numerous kinds of bacteria. Abnormal flora in the GI tract can result in a number of harmful conditions that affect the immune system.

- *Immune suppression.* The immune system can become so weakened that it cannot mount an adequate defense to fight off common illness. This occurs in people with cancer and AIDS but can also result from everyday stress. Stress, for example, has been found to specifically lower the level of protective antibodies through the effects of stress hormones.

- *Lower level of protective antibodies.* For example, levels of antibodies in the intestinal tract, secretory IgA (SIgA), are frequently either suppressed or exaggerated in dysbiosis. In hyperimmune states, as with certain parasitic infections, food allergies, or autoimmune states, levels of SIgA are often increased. (See chapter 2 for more about the role of antibodies.) Treatment of this condition is accomplished by correcting the underlying condition. In situations in which the SIgA is depressed, it may be stimulated through the use of vitamin A and zinc supplements, licorice root exact, or flora supplements such as *Saccharomyces boulardii.*[22,23,24,25,26]

- *Sensitivity and inflammation.* Overreactions and hyper-responsiveness to normal stimuli can develop. This often occurs in cases of asthma, migraine, or food allergies. When the immune system overreacts, it may begin to deplete immune reserves of the body but could also cause responses that injure the tissue through excessive inflammation and the exaggeration of other normally effective defenses.

- *Autoimmune reactions.* A malfunctioning immune system can cause autoimmune reactions, when antibodies become targeted against our own tissues as in rheumatoid arthritis or lupus. In any of these situations, the end result is the same — abnormal body defenses can lead to dysbiosis and can deplete vital immune defenses.

Approaches to Treatment

The diagnosis of dysbiosis centers on several approaches:

- A careful history and physical exam
- An analysis of digestive efficiency
- A specific test called a comprehensive digestive stool analysis (C.D.S.A.)
- Antibody or stool testing for yeast, bacteria, and parasites
- Breath testing for bacterial overgrowth

The ease of treating dysbiosis depends on the strength of our immunity, what we do to improve the integrity of the digestive tract, our nutritional status, and the severity of the infection or overgrowth. In the management of dysbiosis, it is important to treat the underlying problem in the digestive tract whenever possible so that it does not perpetuate the problem. As a result, in situations where there is a severe underlying disease such as AIDS, cancer, or Crohn's disease, the dysbiosis may be impossible to fully correct and may be only partially improved.

In general, restoring the integrity of the digestive tract means carefully evaluating all the possible causes and then finding ways to eliminate them. In the meantime, we can make efforts to manage the dysbiosis by:

- Replenishing the normal microflora
- Providing nutrients that will support healing of the intestinal mucosa
- Reducing toxic exposures
- Supporting normal production of antibodies in the digestive tract

The vitality of the cells in the digestive tract are important in maintaining our resistance. That resistance is also a powerful determinant that controls which microflora can survive. Nutritional support for the gut lining is necessary to maintain our most effective defense mechanisms.[27,28,29,30,31] This support can be provided through nutrients such as:

- A good daily multiple vitamin and mineral supplement
- Supplemental vitamin A and C
- L-glutamine, phosphatidyl choline, and gammaoryzanol
- Essential fatty acids (such as Barlean's flaxseed oil or a high-grade fish oil with gamma linolenic acid or GLA)
- Bioflavinoids (especially quercitin)
- A variety of antioxidants (such as coenzyme Q10, alpha lipoic acid, glutathione, and ginkgo biloba)
- Probiotic supplements to restore flora
- Prebiotic supplements to nourish flora growth
- Colostrum and transfer factor (its protective component) to support general immunity
- Monolauren (lauric acid), which can inhibit the growth of viruses
- Organic foods, especially vegetable juices
- Minimization of toxic exposures

It's also important to keep in mind that dysbiosis is not a disease per se. As a matter of fact, dysbiosis is frequently found in patients who have no specific symptoms, though they often have a vague sense of not feeling well. The presence of disturbed gut ecology is clearly an abnormal finding. It is important information that serves as a warning that something is wrong, even though there are not yet symptoms of disease. It may be a signal that our immune defenses have been compromised or breeched in some way, reflecting the need to restore the competence of the system.

ᘒ

Len Saputo, M.D., is founder and director of the Health-Medicine Forum, a network of more than three thousand health-care professionals that provides information on complementary and alternative medicine for both health-care professionals and a broad public audience. Dr. Saputo is also medical director of the Health Medicine Institute in Walnut Creek, California. Patient services and consultations can be arranged by calling (925) 937-9550.

Notes

1. P. Brandtzaeg, "Development and Basic Mechanisms of Human Gut Immunity," *Nutritional Review* 56, no. 1 (1998): S5–S18.

2. B. A. Araneo et al., "Problems and Priorities for Controlling Opportunistic Pathogens with New Antimicrobial Strategies: An Overview of the Current Literature," *Zentralblatt für Bacteriologie und Hygiene* 283 (1996) 431–465.

3. Great Smokies Diagnostic Laboratory (GSDL), *Comprehensive Diagnostic Stool Analysis Application Guide,* (Asheville, N.C.: GSDL, 1998).

4. R. D. Inman, "Antigens, the Gastrointestinal Tract, and Arthritis," *Rheumatic Dis Clin* NA 17, no. 2 (1991): 309–321.

5. Z. Kassarjian and R. M. Rusell, "Hypochlorhydria: a Factor in Nutrition," *Annual Review of Nutrition* 9 (1989): 271–285.

6. S. P. Borriello, "Gastrointestinal Microflora." In R. Caprilli and A. Torsoli, eds. *Coloproctology: Basic Knowledge for Clinical Practice* (Rome: International University Press, 1990).

7. R. Grubb, T. Midtvedt et al., "The Regulatory and Protective Role of the Normal Microflora," *Proceedings of the 5th Bengt E. Gustafsson Symposium,* Stockholm, Sweden, June 1–4, 1988.

8. G. Latella and R. Caprilli, "Metabolism of Large Bowel Mucosa in Health and Disease," *Int J Colorect Dis.* 6 (1991): 127–132.

9. L. Galland and S. Barrie, "Intestinal Dysbiosis and the Causes of Disease," *J Advancement Medicine* 6 (1993): 67–82.

10. C. Galperin and M. E. Gershwin, "Immunopathogenesis of Gastro-intestinal and Hepatobiliary Diseases," *Journal of the American Medical Association* 278, no. 22 (1997): 1946–1955.

11. See note 9 above.

12. N. Delzenne, G. R. Gibson, and M. Roberfroid, "The Biochemistry of Oligofructose, a Nondigestible Fiber: An Approach to Calculate Its Caloric Value," *Nutrition Reviews* 51, no. 5 (1993): 137–146. Also, see notes 3 and 9 above.

13. See notes 3 and 9 above.

14. See notes 3 and 9 above.

15. B. R. Goldin, "The Metabolism of the Intestinal Microflora and its Relationship to Dietary Fat, Colon and Breast Cancer." In *Dietary Fat and Cancer* (New York: Alan R. Liss, 1986), pp. 655–685.

16. S. N. Lichtman et al., "Hepatic Injury Associated with Small Bowel Bacterial Overgrowth in Rats Is Prevented by Metronidazole and Tetracycline," *Gastroenterology* 100, no. 2 (1991): 513–519.

17. M. Kirsch, "Bacterial Overgrowth," *American Journal of Gastroenterology* 85 (1990): 31–37. Also, see notes 3 and 15 above.

18. See notes 3 and 9 above.

19. W. E. Smalley and M. R. Griffin, "The Risks and Costs of Upper Gastrointestinal Disease Attributable to NSAIDs," *Gastroenterol Clin AN* 25, no. 2 (1996): 373–396.

20. W. E. Whitehead, "The Disturbed Psyche and Irritable Gut," *European Journal of Gastroenterology and Hepatology* 6, no. 6 (1994): 483–488.

21. E. A. Mayer, "The Sensitive and Reactive Gut," *European Journal of Gastroenterology and Hepatology* 6, no. 6 (1994): 470–477.

22. C. M. Surawicz et al., "Treatment of Recurrent Clostridium difficile colitis with Vancomycin and Saccharomyces boulardii," *American Journal of Gastroenterology* 84, no. 10 (1989): 1285–1287.

23. I. R. Rowland, C. J. Rumney, J. T. Coutts et al., "Effect of Bifidobacterium Longum and Inulin on Gut Bacterial Metabolism and Carcinogen-Induced Aberrant Crypt Foci in Rats," *Carcinogenesis* 19, no. 2 (1998): 281–285.

24. H. Majamaa and E. Isolauri, "Probiotics: A Novel Approach in the Management of Food Allergy," *J Allergy Clin Immunol* 99 (1997): 179–185.

25. J. Singh, R. Hamid, and B. S. Reddy, "Dietary Fish Oil Inhibits the Expression of Farnesyl Protein Transferase and Colon Tumor Development in Rodents," *Carcingogenesis* 19, no. 6 (1998): 985–989.

26. J. Sakar, N. N. Gangopadhyay, and Z. Moldoveanu et al., "Vitamin A Is

Required for Regulation of Polymeric Immunoglobulin Receptor Expression by Interleukin-4 and Interferon-g in a Human Intestinal Epithelial Cell Line," *Journal of Nutrition* 128 (1998): 1063–1069.

27. R. R. van der Hulst et al., "Glutamine and the Preservation of Gut Integrity," *The Lancet* 341, no. 8875 (1993): 1363–1365.

28. E. Agostinelli, E. Przybytkowski, and D. A. Averill-Bates, "Glucose, Glutathione, and Cellular Response to Spermine Oxidation Products," *Free Rad Biol Med* 20, no. 5 (1996): 649–656.

29. L. da Silva, T. Tsushida, and J. Terao, "Inhibition of Mammalian 15-lipoxygenase-dependent Lipid Perioxidation in Low-density Lipoprotein by Quercetin and Quercetin Monoglucosides," *Arch Biochem Biophys* 349, no. 2 (1998): 313–320.

30. C. Rukmini and T. C. Raghuram, "Nutritional and Biochemical Aspects of the Hypolipidemic Action of Rice Bran Oil: A Review," *Journal of the American College of Nutrition* 10, no. 6 (1991): 593–601.

31. J. Bustamante, J. K. Lodge, L. Marcocci et al., "Alpha-Lipoic Acid in Liver Metabolism and Disease," *Free Radical Biology and Medicine* 24, no. 6 (1998): 1023–1039. Also, see notes 22, 23, 24, 25, 26 above.

CHAPTER EIGHT

Eating Your Way to Health

Jerry Stine, N.C.

One of the most important influences on our health, minute to minute, is the stability of our blood sugar. When we refer to blood sugar, we are referring to the levels of glucose in the blood. Glucose is one of the primary sources of fuel and energy for the body. Most of us are all too familiar with the feeling we get when we skip a meal and our blood sugar level falls too low. At times like this, our energy level may drop drastically. Some people are also prone to anger or irritability and others tend toward depression. Some experience a loss of concentration, a state that isn't alleviated until they eat something.

Blood Sugar and the Immune System

Most of us don't think of our blood sugar as a powerful regulator of immune function. But blood sugar can affect immunity in a number of important ways:

- *Lower levels of white blood cells* have been associated with a diet high in sugar.[1]
- *The overgrowth of yeast or bacteria* can also result from

eating too many starches and sweets, since carbohydrates are the preferred food of many microbes.[2]

- *Impaired immune function* can result from internal chain reactions that involve insulin and other hormones. This stress can inhibit antibody production.[3]

The stability of our blood sugar has a wide range of effects on:

- Moods
- Mental clarity
- Energy
- Allergic sensitivities
- Metabolism
- Weight
- Potential for diabetes
- Heart health

Jim was a competitive marathon runner. At thirty-five, he was also a busy professional with a wife and young children. In preparing for races, he found that if he trained thoroughly enough to be competitive, he caught every cold or flu his children brought home from school, causing him to miss work. When he didn't train that hard, he wasn't as susceptible, but then he wasn't well prepared for the race. He was anxious to resolve this dilemma — running was important to him, and he was one of the top fifty runners in the state.

Like many of us, he had never paid much attention to his diet or eating on a schedule. In our nutritional counseling sessions, we focused on improving both athletic function and immune response, so that Jim could train to his competitive level and stay healthy. His choice of foods was an issue, because as a runner, he believed he had to eat a diet high in carbohydrates. It took a while for him to become convinced that "carbo loading" was not always the best strategy, particularly in his case.

Through experience, he found that when he reduced his carbohydrate intake, he stopped getting sick. He made it a point to include reasonable levels of protein and fat in his diet and to eat at regular intervals. He was surprised and pleased to find that his immune function improved, and so did his running.

Maintaining stable blood sugar (glucose) is simpler than you would think. It involves just three steps:

1. *Eating the right foods.* Foods that release glucose slowly don't cause drastic highs and lows in blood sugar level.
2. *Finding food options you really enjoy* that are also good for you.
3. *Ideally, having a regular eating schedule,* eating every four or five hours. That may mean just a piece of fruit and some nuts or a protein shake. The idea is to provide the body with a consistent supply of nutrients.

Why Steady Blood Sugar Matters

Blood sugar (glucose) is one of our primary sources of fuel. Most people find that their performance and sense of well-being are improved by having a steady source of energy — stable blood sugar. But many of us tend to eat too many sweet and starchy foods — simple carbohydrates. This has resulted from the modern lifestyle centered on junk food, fast food, and low-fat diets.[4] High-carbohydrate diets can cause health problems, because it's more difficult to maintain consistent blood sugar and energy with a diet that's heavy in simple starches.[5,6,7,8]

Major research has found that diet and poor blood sugar regulation are important risk factors for adult-onset diabetes — Type 2 diabetes.[9] This condition currently affects more than 15 million Americans.[10] A diet low in sugars and starches can often help to prevent the onset of diabetes and is also appropriate for those who are already diabetic. Research also links high carbohydrate intake with conditions such as obesity, high cholesterol and triglycerides, and heart disease.[11] This is a little confusing, because we tend to think of high cholesterol and heart disease as the result of a high-fat diet.[12,13] But the carbohydrate connection to these diseases has been confirmed in some of the most extensive research ever conducted.[14] On the other hand, a low-starch diet has been found beneficial in:

Lowering stress on the body. Rapid changes in blood sugar are a major stress on many crucial systems. Maintaining stable blood sugar can minimize this stress.

Improving health and chronic conditions. Drastic highs and lows in blood sugar can cause immediate problems, including fatigue, mood swings, difficulty concentrating, or insomnia. Over time, it can be a major factor in weight gain, digestive disorders, or chronic depression.

Cutting the risk of disease. Over a lifetime, poor regulation of blood sugar has been linked to obesity, cholesterol problems, heart disease and stroke, diabetes, and the serious disorders that can result from diabetes.[15]

Avoiding weight gain. Since obesity has been linked to both diabetes and heart disease, it is an important health issue.[16] It's much easier to maintain the weight we would like with this style of eating. It is a highly effective tool for natural weight loss.[17]

Supporting healing. Ensuring a steady, reliable source of energy can support the healing process. Correcting this issue in our diet is one of the most important things we can do.

Promoting greater alertness and energy. It's especially important that the brain have a steady supply of glucose.

Improving athletic performance. If you have an athletic interest, this style of eating substantially improves endurance and recovery from intense physical activity.[18]

How It Works and Why It Matters

We can avoid dramatic highs and lows in our energy and mood by choosing foods that encourage stable blood sugar. The key is to eat slow-burning carbohydrates — foods that are broken down gradually — to provide the body with a steady source of nourishment. This means foods such as nuts, popcorn, oatmeal, or sweet potatoes. In contrast, refined sugars and starches are processed too rapidly in the body because they are already partially broken down due to manufacturing. Soon after we eat them, they are quickly absorbed into the bloodstream. As a result, they raise our blood sugar too quickly. This is not only true of foods containing sugar and sweeteners but also of foods made with refined flour such as breads or pastries.

Refined sugars and simple starches are so common in our modern diet that many people experience blood sugar highs and lows every day. When blood sugar (glucoses) is elevated too high, the body is forced to bring the levels down. To cope with high blood sugar, the body releases excessive amounts of insulin, a natural hormone. This brings the blood sugar back to normal levels, but at a price. The body must dispose of it. So some of the blood sugar is expended as energy — remember that energy rush you get right after you eat sugar? And some is stored or converted into fat.

Research has shown that this process is one of the primary causes of excess weight gain. This is also a form of metabolic stress. If we can avoid these rapid increases in blood sugar (and insulin) we can eliminate a major source of stress on the body.

A Quick Guide to the Index

You can copy this chart and carry it in your wallet or purse.

Eating Healthy Made Simple	
Fresh Fruit	**Healthy Starches**
• Berries like blueberries, strawberries, blackberries, and raspberries • Stone fruits such as peaches, plums, and cherries • Apples and pears • Citrus fruits such as oranges and grapefruit • Mangos and kiwi fruit • Eat fruit rather than drinking juice; juices tend to be very sweet, because they are so concentrated.	• Popcorn • Oatmeal, brown rice, and wild rice • Whole-wheat pita bread, tortillas, and chapattis • Sweet potatoes and yams • Pintos and lima beans • Black, kidney, and butter beans
Best Vegetables	**Quality Protein**
• Lettuces, spinach, cilantro, parsleys • Tomatoes • Cucumbers • Leafy green vegetables for cooking: dandelion, chard, and kale • Celery, cabbage, and bok choy • Peas, green beans, and peppers • Asparagus, broccoli, and brussels sprouts • Summer squashes, including zucchini and yellow squash	(Protein usually does not trigger insulin production.) • Unsweetened or lightly sweetened dairy products as tolerated: yogurt, kefir, cheeses, cream cheese, and cottage cheese • Soy and tofu products • Nuts of all types • Eggs • Nutrition bars and protein powders, if low in carbohydrates and high in protein. Eat them in moderation and drink lots of water. • Meat, poultry, and fish

Reproduced with permission. *The Pocket Index.* Nancy Faass, M.S.W., M.P.H., © 2001.

Eating by the Index

One of the easiest ways to eat healthy is to select foods based on their rating on the Glycemic Index. Most people are pleasantly surprised to learn which of their favorite foods are also good for them.

The Glycemic Index is based on scientific research. It's the diet that provides the basis for *The Zone, Sugar Busters!,* Dr. Andrew Weil's *Eating Well for Optimum Health,* and *The Formula.* Maintaining stable blood sugar is also described as glycemic control — referring to glucose (blood sugar). The Index is simply a way of rating foods, based on how much they increase blood sugar and how rapidly it increases. Foods that have a high number on the Index (55 to 150) tend to cause very rapid increases in blood sugar. This happens with foods that are very sweet like desserts or very starchy like baked potatoes. Foods with a high number on the Index also include those made from refined grains like white bread or breakfast cereal that metabolize quickly into glucose. It's helpful to read the Index, because some foods are more problematic than we realize. Surprisingly, rice cakes, for example, are high on the Index.

Foods that break down into glucose more slowly have a lower rating on the Index. Those at 55 or below are either metabolized slower or contain fewer natural sugars. That avoids stressful, drastic changes in blood sugar levels. Again, using the Index involves just three steps:

1. Getting to know the Index.
2. Using it to plan your meals and grocery list.
3. Developing a schedule, so you don't go too long without something to eat.

The Glycemic Index

Foods that are rated at 55 or below are easier for your body to handle.[19] Minimize those above 55 because they trigger insulin.

Foods That Trigger Insulin

Grains, Breads, Cereals, and Vegetables

White bread and baked potatoes	95
Instant rice	90
Cooked carrots	85
French fries, pretzels, rice cakes	80
Corn flakes, corn on the cob	75
Frozen or canned corn	75
Plain bagels	75
Crackers, graham crackers	75
White-flour products, puffed wheat	75
Sweetened cereals	75
White rice, taco shells, beets	70
Spaghetti	60

Sweeteners, Fruits, and Dairy Products

Maltose	105 to 150
Glucose	100
Raisins	95
Honey, refined sugar	75
Watermelon, dried apricots	70
Pineapple	65
Ice cream, ripe bananas	60

The Glycemic Index
Foods That Don't Trigger Insulin

Starches and Vegetables

Oatmeal, brown rice, wild rice	55
Sweet potatoes, popcorn, whole wheat pita bread	55
Yams	50
Green beans, green peas	45
Pinto beans, lima beans	40
Black beans, kidneys, butter beans	30
Nuts	30 to 15
Artichokes	25
Asparagus	20
Tomatoes	15
Green vegetables	15

Fruit and Dairy Products

Mango, kiwi	50
Pears	45
Peaches, plums, apples, oranges	40
Yogurt, with fruit	35+
Milk, whole	30+
Milk, skimmed	30
Cherries, grapefruit	25
Yogurt, plain, no sweetener	15

Planning Balanced Menus

The ratio of nutrients in this diet is typically 40–30–30: 40 percent carbohydrates, 30 percent protein, and 30 percent fats.[20] This is the same ratio used in *The Zone* diet[21] and in *The Formula.*[22] In these diets, every meal is built around low-starch vegetables and high-quality protein. A balanced diet consists of:

40 percent carbohydrates, chosen from fruits and vegetables on the index that are rated at 55 or below. Portion size: about one to two cups of vegetables. You usually don't have to measure out portions as carefully as you would if you were on a diet, because these foods don't tend to cause weight gain. If you want to include starches high on the index, they should not make up more than one-fourth of your carbohydrates at any given meal.

30 percent proteins, that is, three to five ounces of quality protein, depending on your body size and how active you are. The choice of protein varies from one person to another and can be adapted to a vegetarian diet (including dairy and eggs) or vegan diet (nuts, tofu, and soy).

Quality proteins include:
- Dairy
- Eggs
- Nuts
- Protein powders and bars
- Soy and tofu
- Poultry and fish
- Meat

30 percent fat. Good sources of fat include cold-pressed flaxseed, olive oil, safflower, and sunflower oil. Typical servings are $\frac{1}{2}$ to 1 teaspoon of oil per meal, which can be taken as salad dressing.

Applying the Index

When we get hungry, that means we've waited too long to eat and our blood sugar is already beginning to drop. We don't have to eat very much to keep blood sugar steady — in fact, it's not desirable to eat large meals. For people who tend to become hypo-glycemic, it is especially important to have three meals a day and two snacks between meals.

For those of us who are rushed in the morning, breakfast need not involve cooking at all. It could just mean having a pro-tein shake; fruit and cheese; a tuna fish sandwich; or unsweetened yogurt. In general, you don't want to go more than four or five hours without eating. Snacks may be eaten an hour or two before meals — this is another way to prevent overeating at mealtime.

- *Individualizing your diet.* The Index is easy for most people to learn. It may take a month or two to become accustomed to this style of eating. Give yourself permis-sion to adapt gradually. Remember, one of the keys is substitution — replacing foods high on the Index with favorite foods that are low on the Index. For example, have cherries or a peach instead of a banana or raisins.
- *Cut cravings.* Using the Index successfully often involves finding ways to decrease cravings for sweets or starches. See *The Zone* and *The Diet Cure* for additional sugges-tions. Some of the most effective approaches include:

  * Increasing your water intake (see chapter 4)
  * Eating half an apple for dessert
  * Using the French approach — for dessert serve cheeses, salads, or nuts and wine (like Gorgon-zola and walnuts with port)
  * Taking extra vitamin C, the buffered form
  * Taking chromium, a mineral supplement, one dose (200 mcg) on an empty stomach, first thing in the morning (usually well tolerated)

Dining Out

Restaurant meals typically consist of a lot of protein and a lot of starch — for example, a baked potato and a basket of rolls, or pasta and French bread, or a large serving of white rice. The vegetables are often served in small amounts. Keeping blood sugar steady can be achieved by reversing these proportions. Emphasize the vegetables, and just eat a smaller portion of the starch. Say, "No thank you" to at least one of the starches in advance, to avoid temptation and waste. If your willpower is stretched thin, dish up what you want before the meal begins and send back the rest so you won't be tempted to overeat.

To find food that adapts well to this style of eating, plan ahead and make conscious choices when you dine out.[23] Some cuisines work well with this diet:

- Chinese or Thai cooking often offers a good balance with lots of vegetables and moderate protein. Cut down significantly on the rice or noodles, and avoid sweet-and-sour sauces.
- Green salads with grilled chicken are widely available.
- Fish with a salad or vegetables is a good choice.
- Specialty dishes such as fajitas or antipasto that are mainly vegetables and protein are also a good choice.
- Burritos or tacos work well, if you go easy on the beans and rice.
- Nouvelle or Continental cuisine frequently includes great vegetable dishes (be intelligent about the dessert course).

When you're cooking at home, plan ahead so you have leftovers for breakfast and lunch the next day, which really simplifies your routine.

Cheating on the Diet

What can we do about dessert, that special wedding cake or the sweets served at birthdays, holidays, picnics, and other celebrations? When we indulge, we may find ourselves bounced around emotionally — hyper, then depressed, and eventually feeling shaky. It's okay to indulge occasionally, as long as you don't do it too frequently and your reactions aren't too severe. You can avoid a low drop in blood sugar by eating a balanced snack about forty-five minutes to an hour after you eat something really sweet. The snack should include protein, which usually stabilizes blood sugar, and carbohydrates low on the Index. The slower-burning nourishment of the protein tends to sustain the blood sugar, avoiding that blood-sugar roller coaster that can be so depressing.

When Bob was first cleaning up his diet, one thing he didn't have the willpower to give up was root beer. He thought about it all the time, and craved it, and it became one of the few items that was really a problem for him. This was odd, because beforehand he wouldn't have thought of root beer as a favorite beverage. It just surfaced as something he craved. So he let himself have it once a week. His reaction was so dramatic (and so negative) that eventually he stopped wanting it, because every time he indulged, it made him sick. Finally he stopped craving it altogether. Note: This approach only works if your diet is really clean. Otherwise, the symptoms won't show up in the midst of many dietary transgressions.

More Benefits of Using the Index

Following the Glycemic Index can help you reap many significant health benefits.

- *Better digestion.* Eating foods that aren't too sweet or starchy leads to improved digestive health. It also automatically addresses the issues important in food combining. One of the main issues in food combining is that too much sugar or sweet food causes the stomach to empty into the small intestine too soon. When this happens, it means that the first important step of digestion has been completely omitted. This can cause the sense of bloating or indigestion and eventually contribute to allergies or overgrowth.[24]

- *Fewer allergies.* When food passes through the GI tract undigested, it sets the stage for allergies. It can trigger a condition called leaky-gut syndrome, in which large food molecules pass into the bloodstream. This puts a burden on the liver. It also encourages overgrowth and food sensitivities or intolerances, because these undigested food molecules may be viewed by the immune system as foreign substances.[25] The response might be experienced as anything from very subtle symptoms to severe reactions.[26]

- *Ability to identify hidden food allergies.* As you become skilled at using the diet, these stresses on your body will be reduced. At this point, allergies or food sensitivities may become more apparent as other symptoms begin to decrease. You'll be able to see how different foods affect you, so you can individualize your diet, adapted from the suggestions on the Index.

- *Protecting beneficial flora.* Sweets and starches create an environment that tends to encourage the overgrowth of microbes. When there is an overgrowth of yeast such as candida or harmful bacteria, the good flora can be crowded out. Eating a diet moderate in carbohydrates encourages healthy flora.[27] (See chapter 7 for more information about flora and digestion.)

- *Cutting the risk of diabetes.* Once we begin eating a glycemic-controlled diet, a massive stress is removed from the body. This type of diet is called "insulin-sparing," because foods rated at 55 and below on the Index do not call up as much insulin. When you eat a meal low in starches and sugars, your pancreas does not need to produce as much insulin. However, if the liver and the pancreas lose their ability to regulate insulin, diabetes results.[28]

• *Inner balance.* The tendency toward inflammation is also minimized. When blood sugar levels get too high, a whole series of defenses in the immune system are called into play, which can result in inflammation. Keep in mind that blood sugar doesn't just affect one system. All systems of the body are affected by blood sugar and insulin levels, and there is an interrelationship between systems, including the nervous system, the hormones, and immune function.[29]

Martha came to me with a variety of complaints, including poor energy and some memory loss. However, the main thing that motivated her to seek nutritional counseling was that she was getting sick too often. She had a cold or the flu almost every month. Even worse, the illnesses were quite severe; when she got sick, she had a very tangible sense of vulnerability. Although she was in her mid-sixties, she had never experienced anything like that before, and it frightened her.

Once she began a diet that was moderate in starches and low in sugars, her susceptibility to colds and flu declined dramatically. We stayed in contact over the course of a year, and during that time, she was sick only once.

Eating Well and Stronger Immunity

This type of approach provides a sound basis for good immune function. Glycemic control is one of the few things that is usually within our reach. We can't control our genetics. Many exposures to environmental toxins and stress are unavoidable. But most of us have the opportunity to choose the foods we eat. The Index applies to anyone who wants to maintain or improve their health. It is also relevant to those with a health issue, whether it is fatigue, sleep problems, mood swings, difficulty with concentration, allergies, digestive disorders, stress, or any type of immune dysfunction. The most important thing I can tell you about diet is to learn how to use the Index to maintain stable blood sugar. Then apply this approach on a consistent basis in your day-to-day life to provide you with a steady supply of nourishment and energy.

A Public-Service Announcement from Your Pancreas

Hi there,

This is your Pancreas speaking. I know we haven't communicated in a while, what with you being all busy at work and stuff, but I've been trying to send messages your way that I haven't been feeling so great. I'm glad you're finally noticing me, because I was this close to just giving up. Is this really the way we wanted to go?

Please take better care of me. Enough with the donuts and French fries, already. I just can't cope with all the junk you put in your system. And while I've got your attention, another thing — please eat real food, not just anything that costs less than a dollar and comes wrapped in a piece of paper. Processing that stuff really takes it out of me. I want you to be healthy because without you, I'm nothing.

Yours,

Pancreas

P.S. Your Liver sends his regards also, and says that if you keep messing with him like this, he's going to make you sorry for the rest of your life. If you wear us both out, the game's over.

Reprinted courtesy of the author, Dan Tram Nguyen, Van Nuys, California, © 2001.

❧

Jerry Stine, N.C. is a nutritional consultant and the director of the Lifespan Institute, which he founded in 1987 to develop advanced life-extension and performance-enhancement programs. He also founded and directed Health Evaluations, a nonprofit research group with a nutritional consulting clinic and research lab. For the past eight years, he has been an independent nutritional counselor with an active private practice and serves as consultant for several respected vitamin manufacturers. The Lifespan Institute applies functional nutrition concepts with an anti-aging emphasis, providing individual nutritional consultations by phone. Consultations utilize the latest functional testing, including evaluations for allergies, adrenal function, and nutritional status. Lifespan Institute can be reached at (415) 479-3552.

Notes

1. L. Ketikangas-Jarvinene, K. Raikkonen, A. Hautanenen, and H. Adlercreutz, "Vital Exhaustion, Anger Expression, and Pituitary and Adrenocortical Hormones: Implications for the Insulin Resistance Syndrome," *Athroscler ThromboVasc Biol.* 16, no. 2 (1996): 275–280. Also, see D. S. Kelly, and A. Bendick, "Essential Nutrients and Immunologic Functions." *American Journal of Clinical Nutrition* 63, no. 6 (June 1996): 994S–996S.

2. Great Smokies Diagnostic Laboratory (GSDL), *Comprehensive Digestive Stool Analysis Application Guide,* (Asheville, N.C.: GSDL, 1998).

3. J. Lincinio, P. W. Gold, and M. L. Wong, "A Molecular Mechanism for Stress-Induced Alterations in Susceptibility to Disease," *The Lancet* 346 (1995): 104–106.

4. E. Schlosser, *Fast Food Nation* (New York: Houghton Mifflin, 2001).

5. B. Sears, *The Zone* (New York: ReganBooks, 1995).

6. H. Steward et al., *Sugar Busters* (New York: Ballantine, 1998).

7. A. Weil, *Eating Well for Optimum Health* (New York: Random House, 2000).

8. G. and J. Daoust, *The Formula* (New York: Ballantine, 2001).

9. W. B. Kannel, "The Framingham Study: Its 50-Year Legacy and Future Promise," *Journal of Athersoclerosis and Thrombosis* 6, no. 2 (2000): 60–66.

10. NIH Publication No. 99-3892, National Institute of Diabetes and Digestive and Kidney Diseases, March 1999. Website www.niddk.nih.gov/health/dia betes/pubs/dmstats/dmstats.htm#prev, accessed August 9, 2001.

11. See notes 9 and 10 above.

12. S. Liu, W. C. Willett, and M. J. Stamfer et al., "A Prospective Study of Dietary Glycemic Load, Carbohydrate Intake, and Risk of Coronary Heart Disease in Women," *American Journal of Clinical Nutrition* 71, no. 6 (2000): 1455–1561. Also, see note 9.

13. A. K. Kant, A. Schatzkin, B. I. Braubard et al., "A Prospective Study of Diet Quality and Mortality in Women," *Journal of the American Medical Association* 283, no. 16 (2000): 2109–2115.

14. See note 9 above.

15. See notes 10 and 13 above.

16. See note 12 above.

17. See notes 5, 6, 7, and 8 above.

18. See note 5 above.

19. See notes 6 and 8 above.

20. G. and J. Daoust, *40-30-30: Fat Burning Nutrition* (Del Mar, Calif.: Wharton Publishing, 1996).

21. See note 5 above.

22. See note 8 above.

23. E. Haas, *Staying Healthy Shopper's Guide* (Berkeley, Calif.: Celestial Arts Press, 1999).

24. E. Haas, *Staying Healthy with Nutrition* (Berkeley, Calif.: Celestial Arts Press, 1992).

25. See note 25 above.

26. J. Bland, *The 20-Day Rejuvenation Diet Program* (Lincolnwood, Ill.: NTC Publishing, 1999).

27. W. Crook, M.D., *The Yeast Connection Handbook* (Berkeley, Calif.: Professional Books, 1999).

28. L. Tappy and K. Minehira, "New Data and New Concepts on the Role of the Liver in Glucose Homeostasis," *Current Opinion in Clinical Nutrition Metab Care* 4, no. 4 (July 2001): 273–277.

29. T.S. Wolever et al, *The Glucose Revolution: The Authoritative Guide to the Glycemic Index* (New York: Marlowe and Company, 1999). Also, see note 3 above.

CHAPTER NINE

Allergies and Sensitivities

Michael Rosenbaum, M.D.

As a child, Bonnie had recurrent ear infections, and she was usually pale, with dark circles under her eyes. By the age of ten, she seemed to have outgrown the ear infections, although as a teenager she had bouts of hay fever and occasional congestion. However, by the time she reached her thirties, the problems had returned. She felt as if she had a permanent cold, even in the summer: She had a runny nose, stuffiness, and periodic sinus infections. Her tendency to gain weight grew worse, and she became bloated and puffy. Equally distressing, she developed digestive symptoms and was diagnosed with irritable bowel syndrome (IBS).

When she began to develop frequent migraine headaches, she decided that enough was enough and sought out an allergist. Her doctor practiced integrative medicine, combining traditional methods of allergy treatment with new approaches to health and nutrition. He tested her for food allergies, and she scored highly positive to milk, wheat, eggs, and corn (the foods she craved most and ate most often). When the doctor suggested that Sarah eliminate those four foods, she protested: They were her favorites and they would be difficult to give up. He pointed out that these foods tended to be allergenic for a great many of his patients, and that for many, these were also *their* favorite foods.

Once Sarah gathered her resolve and began the elimination diet, she experienced a brief period of withdrawal, which her doctor told her was typical of most all people with allergies. However, as soon as the first three days were over, her congestion began to clear up, and her digestion improved significantly. She lost five pounds of fluid within that first few days, which is typical of food allergy withdrawal. Just by avoiding those foods and substituting others, she found that she began to lose additional unwanted weight more easily, and she didn't even have to cut her calorie intake.

Sarah's doctor pointed out that the longer she could stay on the elimination diet, the better she was likely to feel. She was able to avoid the trigger foods for the required four months. At his suggestion, she began reintroducing the foods into her diet one at a time, about every four days or so. At that point, she found that she tolerated them well and from then on, was able to eat them a couple of times a week without any problems. She also found that she got sick much less often, and when she did, she seemed to bounce back more quickly.

Why be concerned about allergies? Allergies and sensitivities tend to trigger inflammation and other symptoms, so they can place a subtle but constant drain on the immune system. They can also interfere with day-to-day life by causing symptoms that range from congestion to fatigue.

What is less well known is that food allergies and sensitivities are also linked to health problems such as migraines, mood swings, and even neurological symptoms. However, once the offending food is discovered and removed from the diet, there may be rapid improvement, often within the first five days. With allergy treatment, a small investment of time and effort can produce big results. In addition, removing this burden frees up the immune system for stronger defensive efforts when emergencies arise.

What Are Allergies?

The term *allergy* describes an abnormal reaction to substances that the immune system regards as foreign or threatening. A substance that elicits a highly sensitive response in one person may not cause any reaction in another. Substances that cause allergies include pollens, danders, mold, dust, foods, chemicals, and drugs and are called allergens. Allergies can produce symptoms in almost every organ of the body and often masquerade as other diseases. They may affect the skin, eyes, ears, nose, throat, lungs, stomach, bladder, muscles, joints, or even the entire nervous system, including the brain.

By the time most people seek the advice of a doctor, their allergies have existed for some time. Allergies tend to become worse gradually until they cause symptoms that are so uncomfortable that the sufferer feels compelled to do something about them. With food allergies in particular, people tend to become more symptomatic as time goes on.

Causes of Allergies

Allergies are caused by many different factors, alone or in combination.

Heredity. The tendency to have allergies seems to be hereditary. Although parent and child may both have allergies, they may be reactive to different foods or substances.

Infection. It is possible to develop allergic sensitivities after an episode of severe infection, whether viral, bacterial, or fungal.

Chemical exposure. Heavy exposure to pesticides or petrochemicals can also lead to the development of allergic reactions.

Stress. Increased stress, whether emotional or physical, positive (getting married) or negative (getting fired), can play a role in allergies.

Nutrition. Poor nutritional habits contribute to the development of allergies as well as other illnesses.

Immediate and Delayed Allergies

Dr. Alan Levin was one of the first to differentiate between immediate and delayed allergies. In his book, *The Type 1 and 2 Allergy Relief Program,*[1] he describes immediate allergies as Type 1 and delayed allergies as Type 2.

Immediate Allergies: Type 1

Although the symptoms of Type 1 allergies fit the classic pattern of an allergy, they are relatively uncommon — these are *immediate* reactions that may be life threatening. People with Type 1 allergies have instant reactions, are usually well aware of their response, and may carry adrenaline with them in case of a reaction. The foods that typically cause these reactions are shellfish (such as crab, lobster, or shrimp), various types of nuts, cinnamon (used as a spice), and peanuts (actually a type of bean). With immediate Type 1 allergies, the same type of antibody that causes hay fever (IgE) also causes allergies to specific foods. (You can remember the antibody IgE by associating it with E for emergency, although that is not its actual meaning. See chapter 2 for more about the role of antibodies.)

The tendency to Type 1 allergies (IgE associated) is often hereditary. Periodically there are stories in the newspapers about someone suddenly passing out in a restaurant, unable to breath due to anaphylactic shock and having to be taken to a hospital immediately because of something they ate. The cause could be something as innocent as a trace of peanuts in a sauce, but the response is immediate and intense. These are usually Type 1 allergies.

Delayed Allergies: Type 2

Type 2 allergies are gradual reactions, associated with the IgG antibody (think of G for gradual). These responses may also be caused by triggers that are not related to antibodies. Foods such as wheat, for example, have been found to cause responses with long delays — symptoms may not develop for as long as two days after the food has been eaten. Because of the delay in response, it is often much more difficult to diagnose delayed reactions to food, which constitute perhaps 90 percent of the responses reported to allergists. These are cases in which there is no obvious, immediate cause and effect. In addition, there may or may not be a genetic link.

Food Sensitivities

Another category of response is sensitivity to both foods and chemicals, such as food additives and coloring, pesticides, or pollutants. Research suggests that a number of different mechanisms may be associated with food sensitivities. Some of these processes may not be triggered by antibodies at all. Possible causes of delayed food sensitivities include:

- A pattern of faulty digestion described as "leaky-gut syndrome"
- Stimulation of the nervous system, sites in the brain, or receptor nerve cells, with symptoms of confusion, difficulty concentrating, or even attention deficit disorder

- Activity associated with the effects of hormones or neurotransmitters or triggered by certain proteins (such as peptides)

Minimizing Allergies and Sensitivities

The process of treating people for food allergies and sensitivities basically involves discovering the food that triggers the allergy and then eliminating it from their diet. Once people realize how good they feel without their reactive symptoms, it becomes almost effortless for them to give up problematic foods. Of the basic treatments for food allergies, elimination of the offending food is probably the most important and useful approach. The primary approaches to allergy treatment include:

- Elimination of the allergen
- The rotation diet
- Desensitization
- The use of digestive enzymes with meals

The Food Challenge

One of the most effective means of testing for food sensitivities is the home food challenge, often considered the gold standard of testing for food allergies. Although the test is simple and inexpensive, it can provide extremely useful information for detecting and eliminating allergenic foods and the symptoms that can result from eating them.

The first step is to stop eating the major foods suspected of causing symptoms. In response, people usually find that their body goes through a period of withdrawal from these foods, in which they may experience aches, fatigue, or other symptoms. Before testing specific foods, it is important to allow the body to return to balance (homeostasis). Waiting a period of seven days before testing new foods allows for four days of withdrawal and then two to three days for clinical improvement to occur. From the seventh day on, a variety of suspected foods can be gradually reintroduced and monitored, testing them one at a time.

Typically, this test is done at lunchtime. A large serving of one particular food is consumed as the only food in a "monomeal." If there are no obvious symptoms within thirty minutes to an hour, the food can be eaten again, in a serving half the size of the meal. Typically a positive response (indicating an allergy) will occur within three hours of ingesting the sample food. If a reaction doesn't occur on the day of testing, symptoms may be evident on awakening the next morning. People may feel even worse the following day, with symptoms that resemble a hangover. If the reaction is intense and uncharacteristic, it could indicate a delayed food sensitivity.

The food should be tested at a time when you are not working, so you can monitor your reactions carefully and are more likely to notice any symptoms that may occur. Whenever there is a reaction, wait until it has completely subsided before testing another food. If you want to expedite the process, you can take a laxative such as Milk of Magnesia to force the food out of your system completely. Otherwise, you may have to wait two or three days until the symptoms of the first reaction have totally cleared before testing another food. The food challenge is best done when you have enough time and attention.

Unmasking the Allergy

In some cases, allergies and sensitivities tend to trigger food cravings and addictive responses. Taking a medical history for allergies involves identifying the foods patients crave. Often you can predict the foods to which a person is allergic if they say, "You can take anything out of my diet, doctor, but please don't ask me to give up chocolate." The very foods craved the most tend to be the source of the allergy.

Overcoming the Allergy:
What to Do and What Not to Do

When a food is eliminated from the diet, a process of unmasking occurs in which a person may feel worse rather than better.

- *Tolerance.* If we are eating an allergenic food as part of our normal diet, the body may mask the reaction. We may be unaware of any reactivity, and a kind of tolerance can develop toward the food — in fact, this response is described as tolerance. When the food is withdrawn, we may become intolerant of the food, experiencing much greater sensitivity to that particular food.
- *Withdrawal.* It is well documented that allergens can have addictive properties. Someone who is trying to eliminate an allergy may experience a period of withdrawal very similar to that experienced by alcoholics or drug addicts when they stop using a particular substance. This is the initial stage in the process of "unmasking" the allergy. The withdrawal period usually lasts about four days. On one or two of those days, often people crave the very foods that have been removed from their diets and may have uncomfortable symptoms such as aches, pains, diarrhea, a runny nose, or fatigue. That is the unmasking or withdrawal effect.
- *Resensitizing.* During the unmasking period, the person becomes resensitized to the reactive or allergenic food. After the four days of the withdrawal period, the person becomes extra sensitive to this particular food. This period of supersensitivity lasts for about three to four weeks.

When the allergy is unmasked, and the individual becomes sensitive to that food once again, a strong response can be elicited if the food is reintroduced too soon. We may become as sensitive as we would have been as an infant. During that time, when allergic individuals eat the particular food to which they are sensitive, they could have an exaggerated reaction, more intense and extreme than their normal response to the food when they ate it frequently.

It is important to be very strict for the first four weeks, during the unmasking period. If the allergenic food is reintroduced too early in the program, one can become extremely ill. I have had patients who were very careful for two weeks and then cheated on their diet, with uncomfortable consequences. Typically people rationalize this kind of decision: "I've been so good for two weeks, now that I'm invited out to a dinner party, I'll treat myself — after all, it's only one meal." As a result, an exaggerated reaction can occur, which might include any kind of allergic response:

- Mental symptoms such as confusion or difficulty with concentration
- Abdominal discomfort such as nausea, vomiting, or diarrhea
- A skin rash or hives
- Rapid heartbeat
- Extreme fatigue that begins suddenly
- Headache
- Intense muscle aches and pains

The Pulse Test

Another approach to allergy testing is the Pulse Test,[2] developed by Dr. Arthur Coca, a famous allergist at Columbia University in the 1920s. He found that when people with food allergies ate an allergenic food during the initial sensitive period, they usually experienced an increase in their pulse rate of at least twelve beats per minute. This reactivity provides the basis for another type of home testing, the Pulse Test.

The process involves establishing a baseline pulse, taken throughout the day for a period of seven days. People notice that most often they have one particular pulse rate — their baseline. The seven days also serve as the unmasking period in which the foods most likely to trigger sensitivities are removed from the diet. Once a baseline pulse is established, significant changes in pulse are quite apparent when consuming an offending food.

1. To perform the test, the pulse is taken and a small portion of the food is eaten.
2. Then the pulse is checked half an hour later.
3. If the pulse has gone up to least twelve to sixteen beats a minute, that is a sign that the food may be triggering a reaction. That serves as a positive test. A small serving of food will not trigger all the symptoms associated with a monomeal, but some people may experience some symptoms within an hour of ingesting an allergenic food and they usually will within three hours.

Dealing with Reactions

Bicarbonate can often be used by itself to treat an accidental reaction that may result from allergy testing. When feeling unwell after a restaurant meal, consider taking Alka-Seltzer Gold or $\frac{1}{2}$ teaspoon of bicarbonate soda or a mixture of tri-salts (a mixture of sodium, potassium, and calcium, available from compounding pharmacies). This mixture can sometimes dispel the symptoms completely within five minutes.

The Rotation Diet

Some people with serious food allergies or sensitivities find that they can still tolerate many foods as long as they don't eat them daily. By rotating foods every four days, they are able to eat allergenic foods without developing symptoms. The rotation diet offers major benefits: It allows you to minimize your exposure to any one food, and makes it easier to monitor foods and identify those that may be causing reactions.

When people are sensitive to a wide range of foods, it's not enough to simply eliminate one or two foods. The best solution is to eat a varied diet, by rotating many different foods to make sure that no one food is repeated too often and to assure proper nutrition by eating a variety of foods.

1. In a rotation diet, any food that is eaten one day is usually not repeated until four days later.
2. A series of meal plans are developed with foods that are eaten together for day one, day two, day three, or day four.
3. Then the combination of foods from day one is repeated on the fifth day. Day two's combination is repeated on the sixth day and so forth.
4. With this type of planning, you can create menus and meals that include foods and food combinations you enjoy (as long as you can tolerate them).
5. Planning begins with a list of fruits, vegetables, grains and beans, and protein foods.
6. Make sure that whatever is consumed together is always eaten together on that day of the diet.

Another important aspect of these diets is the rotation of food families. The principle here is that foods fall into biological families. For instance, lemons, grapefruit, oranges, and limes are all in the same citrus family. In these cases, foods can be grouped by food family. Lemons and oranges might be eaten on Monday and Friday, but limes and grapefruit would be taken on Wednesday and Sunday. In that way, you can actually eat food in the same family four times in one week.

A Rotation Diet for Severe Allergies

There are a number of ways of organizing a food-rotation diet. People with severe food allergies may need a seven-day rotation; these are people who are still reactive to food on a four-day rotation diet. In one sense the seven-day rotation is easier, because the days of the week never change. What you eat on Monday is always what you eat on Monday. If you require this diet, it can be used to your advantage. For example, you can devise the menu so that you plan special meals for the weekend that feature your favorite foods.

Each day of the week includes the same foods, week to week. However, within that menu, you can vary what you cook tremendously. For example, if Thursday is chicken night, the chicken can be prepared in any of dozens of ways to keep it interesting, as long as the choices of foods and condiments are made with the diet in mind.

Some allergies may be permanent. Foods that trigger these permanent allergies may need to be completely eliminated from the diet. Foods that are tolerated can be eaten on a rotation basis. Generally, most foods can be taken every four days. However, a few specific foods may need to be eaten every seven or eight days, if there is greater sensitivity.

It's helpful to remember that cooked foods are less allergenic than raw foods. Cooked tomato sauce tends to be less allergenic than a raw tomato. The same is true of applesauce and fresh apples. Another basic principle is that people tend to be more allergic to foods in cold weather than in warm weather.

Using Digestive Enzymes

Another theory about food reactivity is that reactions to food may be caused by incomplete digestion and are triggered when partly digested food molecules are absorbed. A solution to this problem is to supplement the body's digestive enzymes with an enzyme product and bicarbonate. The goal is to break down the food more thoroughly. This approach is most helpful to someone whose body doesn't produce enough enzymes or enough bicarbonate. Another theory of food allergy proposes that the problem may involve not only the completeness of digestion but also other types of problems within the digestive tract.

Protein digestive enzymes. By supplementing essential enzymes, you may find that you digest your food better. For dosage, see the manufacturer's recommendation, typically from one to three capsules (depending on the strength of the product), which can be taken toward the end of the meal or fifteen to twenty minutes after the meal.

Bicarbonates. If a little bicarbonate is added after taking enzymes, the enzymes tend to work better. One form of bicarbonate that is used a great deal, because it contains no aspirin, is Alka-Seltzer Gold, a combination of sodium and potassium bicarbonate. The bicarbonate helps the pancreatic enzymes work better by creating the necessary alkaline environment. Bicarbonate soda may also be taken.

Testing and Treatment by an Allergist

There are a number of types of medical testing for food allergies for people who lack the time or inclination to do accurate home challenge testing. One way that physicians frequently test for food allergies is through skin testing. This testing is usually provided in the doctor's office, often by a trained technician under the supervision of the physician. There are a number of different types of skin tests and testing procedures.

Types of Skin Tests

Skin tests for allergies include:

The prick, or scratch test used by most allergists tends to produce inconsistent results (false negatives and false positives). The test findings often don't correlate very well with what we see in the food challenge tests.

Intradermal testing involves injecting the allergen underneath the skin rather than just scratching the skin. This method tends to be more accurate.

Skin testing to measure the degree of individual sensitivity. Another form of skin testing was devised by the famous allergist Dr. Herbert J. Rinkel during the 1940s[3] and further developed by Dr. Joseph Miller in Alabama. The idea here is not just to test reactivity but also to determine the exact level of sensitivity an individual experiences to each specific food, so that a treatment dose or antidote can be individualized for that person. In this type of testing, intradermal skin tests are performed, but a series of varying dilutions are used for each allergenic food. In the testing, two, three, or more injections of each food are given in a different concentration (in dilutions of one to five). At the end of the testing, the antidotes for all the foods causing allergies can be put together into one formula. Injections of the antidote can be given on an individual schedule, depending on the severity of the allergy. Some people take them daily or even several times a day. Others get injections twice a week.

Treating Allergies with Simple Antidotes

Another treatment technique is to give doses of the offending food or substance (the allergen) sublingually. In that case, the doses are usually taken two to three times a day. The length of treatment depends on the individual's needs. The therapy may be given for one or two years, or it may be required indefinitely. People are usually retested about once a year to see if their doses have shifted. This particular technique of testing is used more often by ear-nose-and-throat doctors than by traditional allergists. There is some disagreement regarding the best approaches to treatment. However, innovators in this field such as Drs. Rinkel and Miller reported that this approach has been beneficial to many people with sensitivities.

Food allergies are a common cause of distress for a great many people — yet often go undetected. Typically, the symptoms are not just localized in the nose or throat — they can result in fatigue, muscle aches and pains, and a wide variety of other problems as well. Yet when there are chronic health issues, allergies tend to be something we overlook because there is no obvious cause. Often the unsuspected villains are familiar foods that are consumed every day. So when a chronic condition has not responded to treatment, it is important to evaluate for allergies — this is the piece of the puzzle practitioners consider when everything else fails. Fortunately, these conditions are quite treatable. With the sensitive testing and advanced therapies now available, allergies may be easily detected and usually successfully resolved.

~⤳

Michael Rosenbaum, M.D., of Corte Madera, California, has had an active private practice since 1977 focused on clinical nutrition, immunology, and allergy. He can be reached for consultations on nutritional therapy, allergy treatment, and antiaging medicine, by calling his office at (415) 927-9450.

Notes

1. A. S. Levin and M. Zellerbach, *The Type 1 and 2 Allergy Relief Program* (New York: Berkley Publishing Group, 1986).
2. A. F. Coca, *The Pulse Test: The Secret of Building Your Basic Health* (New York: St. Martin's Press, 1996).
3. H. J. Rinkel et al., *Food Allergy* (The New England Foundation, 1976).

dealing
with toxins

Clearing Toxins for Life
Ellen Cutler, M.D., D.C.

Minimizing Your Exposure to Toxins
Jeffry Anderson, M.D.

CHAPTER TEN

Clearing Toxins for Life

Ellen Cutler, M.D., D.C.

Joseph, a fourteen-year-old diagnosed with asthma, came to see me with his parents, who were concerned that their son's condition was growing worse. They expressed the hope that allergy treatments would improve his situation. Since allergies are known to be a major cause of asthma, I began by reviewing Joseph's diet. I learned that he lived on fast-food lunches such as hot dogs, sausages, and hamburgers, which include food additives, food coloring, and preservatives, as well as soft drinks with a high sugar content. His diet contained few fruits or vegetables, and he almost never ate fresh organic produce, a good source of nutrients and trace minerals. He lacked wholesome, balanced meals.

I encouraged Joseph to begin educating himself about nutrition. After having him fill out a detoxification questionnaire and reviewing the results, I recommended that he take a homeopathic remedy for gentle cleansing. I also discussed with him some diet recommendations, including skipping the soft drinks and, at least three days a week, packing a more healthful school lunch that included a sandwich made with whole-grain bread, a good organic source of protein such as turkey, some vegetable sticks, and spring water.

Joseph agreed to these changes, and, when he returned in three weeks, he looked completely different. His asthma had disappeared, and his acne had improved. He felt more energetic than he had in years, and he reported that he needed less sleep to feel rested. I then began giving him BioSET allergy elimination treatments. Three years later, he no longer requires any type of medication.

The incidence of immune disorders is increasing: Many people all over the world are being diagnosed with various conditions that relate to impaired immunity. I truly believe that we need to reevaluate our lives. That means noticing and repairing the toxic burdens that are imposed on our minds and bodies, reflected in our loss of inner balance.

When toxins assault us or build up in the body, the immune system's capacity to protect us can be overwhelmed. Food allergies, for example, are often the result of those insults. How do we discern the difference between toxicity and food allergies? Initially, it is nearly impossible to do so. That is why the first step I take with my clients is a program of detoxification. Once the body has been detoxified, we can look at the remaining symptoms. Frequently, the problems that persist after detoxification can be correlated with various food allergies and addressed through allergy treatment. It is also important to develop a consistent long-term program that enables the body to periodically detoxify.

This program may involve:

- Changing the way we eat
- Recipes to help get us started
- Foods to avoid
- Exercising
- Detoxifying from trauma and stress
- Minimizing toxic exposure

Changing the Way We Eat

Changing one's diet is a great way to detoxify the body and return it to a state of balance, or homeostasis. One good example of a diet that helps the body to detoxify is the macrobiotic diet. This type of diet stresses eating only foods grown in the area in which you live that are in season. For example, if you live in the northern United States or Canada, you should avoid eating tropical fruits. A macrobiotic diet also includes eating as many whole foods as possible, such as brown rice, millet, whole rye, and foods that have not been refined by any processing, canning, or denaturing. Ideally, these foods should be cooked to preserve their nutrients. Use sea salt instead of table salt, because it contains more minerals. Optimum cooking involves steaming or braising foods rather than boiling or baking them and poaching instead of frying.

The classic macrobiotic diet consists of 50 to 60 percent whole grains, 20 to 30 percent locally grown vegetables, 5 to 10 percent beans and sea vegetables, 5 to 10 percent soups, and 5 percent condiments and other foods. Avoid highly processed foods and sugar, dairy products, and red meat and poultry. Here are some recipes that I enjoy and recommend to my patients.

Favorite Recipes

Miso Soup
Serves 4

2 dried shiitake mushrooms

4 cups filtered or spring water

$\frac{1}{3}$ block firm tofu, cubed

1 tsp. organic toasted sesame oil

3 Tbsp. miso (organic or traditional barley miso, or red miso)

green onions, sliced for garnish

Soak shiitakes in 1 cup of the filtered water for 20 minutes. Remove and slice thinly. Combine soaking water and remaining 3 cups of filtered water, bring it to a boil, and add the shiitakes. Reduce to simmer for 5 minutes. Add the tofu to the stock and heat through. Make a thin paste of miso with the stock, add it to pot, and warm on low for 2 minutes. Garnish with green onions and serve.

Tofu Salad
Serves 2 to 4

1 block firm tofu

3 Tbsp. miso (barley, white, or chickpea miso)

1 to 2 Tbsp. pickled ginger, chopped fine, and its juice

2 tsp. tahini

1 tsp. organic toasted sesame oil

1 stalk celery, diced small

2 green onions, thinly sliced

1 cup chopped sprouts (preferably daikon)

Press the tofu under a weighted plate for 30 minutes to release excess moisture. Blot with towels. Combine the miso with the pickled ginger and add a teaspoon of ginger juice, the tahini, and toasted sesame oil. Crumble the tofu with your hands into large bowl. Add miso mixture and combine thoroughly. Stir in celery, green onions, and sprouts. Spread on toasted whole-grain bread or stuff into a tortilla with lettuce and carrots. (This is one of my favorites.)

Azuki Bean and Winter Squash Stew
Serves 6 to 8

1 $\frac{1}{2}$ cups azuki beans

6 cups filtered water

3 cups winter cubed winter squash

2 tsp. miso (organic barley, red, or brown rice miso)

1 tsp. organic toasted sesame oil

1-inch piece of fresh ginger

Soak the beans overnight. Discard the soaking water, and bring the beans to a boil in 6 cups of filtered water. Lower the heat and pressure cook for 20 minutes, or simmer for 60 minutes on the stove. When the beans are almost tender, add winter squash and simmer for 20 minutes or until the squash is tender. Using some of the bean liquid, dilute the miso. Add the sesame oil and ginger juice (peel and grate the ginger, then, using your hands, squeeze out the juice). Add this to the pot and heat for 5 minutes, stirring occasionally.

Dairy-Free Pesto
Makes approximately $\frac{3}{4}$ cup

1 cup tightly packed fresh basil, leaves only

2 to 4 cloves garlic, peeled

$\frac{1}{4}$ cup fresh parsley, destemmed

$\frac{1}{4}$ cup walnuts or pine nuts, toasted

2 to 4 Tbsp. organic miso (barley, white, or chickpea miso)

$\frac{1}{4}$ to $\frac{1}{2}$ cup extra virgin olive oil

Combine the first 5 ingredients in a blender or food processor. Very slowly trickle the olive oil through top of the machine with the motor running, or if you're using a blender, add a little oil periodically, until the desired consistency is formed. This pesto may be smooth or chunky, according to your liking. Serve with vegetables or stir into soup for a flavorful treat!

Hummus

Serves 2 to 4

1 cup chickpeas, cooked

2 cloves garlic

2 Tbsp. tahini

1 lemon, juiced (1 $\frac{1}{2}$ Tbsp. juice)

Blend all the ingredients in a food processor or blender. Serve as a dip for pita bread, crackers, or veggies, or as a delicious sandwich spread with red onion, lettuce, and tomato.

These are just a few of my favorite recipes. You can find many more in *American Macrobiotic Cuisine* by Meredith McCarty[1] and *Aveline Kushi's Complete Guide to Macrobiotic Cooking.*[2]

Foods to Avoid

General Suggestions

If we want to have a healthy, toxin-free body, it is important to avoid certain foods. Eating as many organic foods as possible and remaining on a balanced diet will help us to perform and function to the best of our ability. I suggest that readers avoid the following items:

- Refined sugars and other refined carbohydrates
- Caffeine. This additive substance inhibits the body's natural ability to detoxify.
- Alcohol. It is also addictive and causes degeneration of our cells.
- Foods and beverages with a high sodium content. A high salt intake can cause a deficiency of potassium, an important mineral for healthy muscles, including the muscles of the heart.
- Artificial sweeteners, food additives, and food coloring
- Foods that have been sprayed with pesticides and fungicides — these foods are potentially carcinogenic and toxic.

Genetically Altered Foods

It is also important to avoid eating any genetically altered foods. These are sometimes called GMOs, for "genetically modified organisms" and are now sold in supermarkets across the country and around the world. In recent years, many grains and produce have been altered to contain elements that fight the growth of bacteria in order to promote longer shelf life.[3] The consequences of gene splicing can be devastating. For people with allergies, GMOs can trigger an allergic response if the food in question contains genes from a food to which they are allergic. When a gene from Brazil nuts was spliced into soybeans to make them taste nuttier, a product was created that has the potential to cause a severe nut allergy. Genetically altered corn has not been approved for human use, because it contains proteins similar to those known to cause allergic reactions.[4]

What's more, these altered foods do not have to be tested for safety and require no labeling to inform you of genetic material added to the original food. GMOs are so widespread that it is likely you are already eating them, unless all the foods you eat are organic. Soybeans and corn have been modified since 1996 with genes from bacteria, viruses, and other sources that are not native to human food. If you are eating anything with corn or soy added to it, you're probably eating GMOs.

There has not been adequate testing to determine the environmental consequences of GMOs. For this reason, we need to lobby Congress for a law that requires all foods containing GMOs to be labeled. Although the F.D.A. claims that GMOs are equivalent to conventional food, there is overwhelming evidence that some of them are potentially very dangerous to our health, and there's a growing concern about the safety of GMOs in this country. In countries where people have protested, there have been changes. For example, in England GMOs are not being used by fast food chains.[5] In the United States, a major baby food company has also stopped using GMOs. If you see signs in supermarkets that say

Genetically Modified Organisms, you will know that the label actually means: This food is unsafe to eat!

Exercising

A systematic program of exercise is essential to detoxification, because it strengthens the cardiovascular system. Lack of exercise causes toxins to build up in our bodies, destroying our homeostasis. Studies have shown that exercise can actually speed up the removal of toxins and waste materials from the cells and increase blood flow that carries nutrients to every cell.[6] Exercise can also lower blood pressure and cholesterol, which helps prevent heart attacks. A consistent program of exercise increases your body temperature, restores lung power, and improves bone structure and muscle flexibility. It can also aid in weight reduction and shorten the duration of allergic reactions. Exercise has many emotional and psychological benefits and can generally improve mental health by:

- Decreasing anger and hostility
- Reducing stress
- Elevating moods with the release of natural biochemicals, endorphins
- Improving mental abilities, memory, and learning potential

Aerobic Exercise

Aerobic activities such as brisk walking, jogging, or swimming, are one of the best forms of exercise. Aerobic exercise should be done for a minimum of thirty to forty-five minutes at least three times a week. To be considered aerobic, an exercise must raise your heartbeat to what is known as the Ideal Exercise Heartbeat Rate per Minute. To calculate this rate, subtract your age from the number 220. When you multiply the resulting figure by 0.6, this should give you your lowest healthy heartbeat rate. When you multiply it by 0.85, you will get your highest healthy heartbeat rate. It is advisable to monitor your pulse while exercising to be certain that you are within the proper heartbeat range. If your heart is racing wildly, you are overdoing it. A good sign that you are exercising at the right intensity is always being able to carry on a conversation during exercise. If you cannot, you are exercising too hard. I have found moderate aerobic exercise done consistently over a longer period of time to be more effective than strenuous exercise in short bursts. Even moderate aerobics encourage the release of endorphins, natural substances secreted by the brain that bring about a feeling of euphoria and well-being.

Running

It is estimated that there are more than 33 million runners in America alone. Running has always been my favorite form of exercise, because it improves lung capacity; strengthens the legs, muscles, and bones; reduces body fat; and improves circulation. I feel an instant positive mood change when I run. Yet running is not something that I, as a chiropractor, have recommended to most of my patients. Since it is a high-impact exercise, running can be a risk for those with a history of knee, hip, or ankle problems or lower back conditions.

If you do choose to run, know that warming up by stretching beforehand is critical to prevent sprains, strains, and tendonitis. Always remember that burning pain in your muscles while exercising and extended cramping afterward are clear indications that your method of exercise is too strenuous.

Swimming

Regular long-distance swimming produces the same benefits as running, cycling, or cross-country skiing. One advantage of swimming is that it can cause you to become fit very rapidly. Exercise in the pool may take the form of swimming laps; running, walking, or jumping in the water; or using a kickboard. The water acts as a giant cushion for these activities, absorbing the shock of the movements and providing low-impact exercise. Because water has more resistance than air, walking or running in water makes your leg muscles, heart, and lungs work hard, even though your speed for these activities will be slower. Water exercise sessions are available at some public pools.

Chlorinated pool water can be a particular threat to asthmatics and those who are sensitive to chlorine. Wear goggles to help protect your eyes. Some swimmers use a nose clip to prevent water from entering the nose. Showering immediately after swimming is always a good idea.

Cycling

Cycling is not a weight-bearing activity and, therefore, it is less stressful to your joints than running. Bicycling can be as beneficial as running, because it increases circulation and the flow of oxygen to your cells and helps to eliminate toxins. Stationary bicycles offer more environmental control and safety than do outdoor bicycles. The best stationary bicycles are those that exercise your arms as well as your legs.

There are a number of other exercise systems that are as effective as aerobic exercises for cleansing and detoxifying. Meditative exercises such as Qigong and yoga address the needs of the body, mind, and spirit. (See chapter 5 for information on a range of gentle exercises, including Qigong and t'ai chi, yoga, and walking.)

Detoxifying from Trauma and Stress

A great deal has been written about trauma, stress, and the suppression of emotions as a source of toxicity and cause of disease. I see this every day in my patients, in everyone from two-year-olds to eighty-year-olds. Since emotional stress has a significant impact on the health of our bodies, our stress must always be acknowledged and addressed.

Our conscious mind might have suppressed and forgotten our psychological traumas, but our subconscious memory and our cells remember. These traumatic memories wear down the body and our immune, endocrine, and nervous systems. Although we often overlook the psychological aspects of toxicity, trauma, or negativity, their impact on our lives is very real. Among the resources for reducing toxicity in our lives, exercise may be one of the most important.

The BioSET Allergy Elimination Treatment also provides a means for clearing these emotional wounds.[7] This, however, is not the kind of treatment that can be done at home. Rather, it needs to be taken under the guidance of a skilled BioSET practitioner.

To avoid the buildup of toxicity through emotional distress, taking preventative measures is crucial. Seek therapy when it is appropriate. Counseling and psychotherapy are helpful as tools for cleansing and de-stressing both our minds and our bodies. I have also used homeopathic Bach flower remedies for emotional trauma, abuse, and stress. Keeping a journal either daily or during times of stress is another great tool to promote emotional health. Recording our happy experiences, as well as our problematic and disturbing ones, is a great technique for evening ourselves out. Writing allows you to be who you really are and gives you the opportunity to say whatever you like.

What goes on in the mind and emotions can influence the body. It is most important to never suppress your feelings; find appropriate venues to release them and build opportunities for release into your life. I have seen people achieve effective emotional detoxification by learning how to cry, to be patient, and to express their emotions and frustrations constructively. Having faith and accepting and forgiving what cannot be changed are also important. I encourage my patients to cultivate an open, peaceful loving existence; to relax and to laugh; to sit and meditate or contemplate nature; to listen to music or to play it. Laughter is another power-ful tool for cleansing and healing. In his book *Anatomy of an Illness,* Norman Cousins discusses the therapeutic benefits of laughter and love.[8] We can access the lighter side of our nature by watching a funny movie, listening to humorous tapes, reading clever books, or by spending time with a young child who makes us smile or laugh.

Minimizing Toxic Exposure

Most of us are assaulted daily by a toxic world — fast-food restau-rants, food additives, a diet of highly processed foods, toxic chemicals, and radiation. The soil is contaminated with pesticides and herbicides, and even our drinking water has become con-taminated with toxic chemicals and microorganisms such as bac-teria and parasites. Industrial wastes have exposed us to harmful substances such as hydrocarbons, phenols, and petrochemicals. (See chapter 11 for more information on minimizing toxins in your environment.)

Other common sources of toxins in everyday life include envi-ronmental factors such as:

- Synthetic toxins like heavy metals and plastics
- Natural toxins such as bacteria, parasites, viruses, fungi, as well as pollens
- Smog and noise
- Electromagnetic energy from high-voltage cables and household electronic devices such as computers, televi-sion, and clock radios
- Geopathic stress from living in a place where the earth's magnetic fields are especially strong
- Household toxins ranging from cleaning products to solvents
- Toxins in our foods, such as coloring, preservatives, and other additives

Internal toxins include:

- Inherited genetic disorders passed from generation to generation
- Poorly digested food
- Stress and emotional trauma

Toxins are also produced or processed within our own body — metabolic wastes that our system can not metabolize and remove such as excess uric acid, free radicals (substances that can cause damage or death to cells), residues of medicinal and recreational drugs, and synthetic hormones such as estrogen and cortisol.

Building Detoxification into Your Daily Life

Detoxification is a moment-to-moment challenge to our personal awareness. There is much that we cannot control in our lives and in the lives of those we love, but there are also many things that we can do. And we must do what we can, for our own sakes and theirs. Keeping ourselves, our families, and our environment as toxin free as possible is an investment in time, and perhaps even in money, but it is well worth the effort. Detoxification is a critical factor in good health, and you will reap many benefits from your efforts.

⌇

Ellen Cutler, M.D., D.C., holds a medical degree from University of California, Los Angeles, and a degree in chiropractic from Western States Chiropractic College in Portland, Oregon. She is the innovator of BioSET, a type of applied acupressure therapy that has been used to successfully treat thousands of people with allergies and related symptoms. She is also founder of BioSET Institute, which can be reached at (877) 927-0741 and on the Web at www.bioset-institute.com.

Notes

1. M. McCarty, *American Macrobiotic Cuisine* (New York: Penguin/Putnam, 1996).
2. A. Kushi, *Aveline Kushi's Complete Guide to Macrobiotic Cooking* (New York: Warner Books, 1989).
3. K. Severson, "Taco Shells Symbol for Frankenfood," *San Francisco Chronicle,* Restaurant Section, September 18, 2000.
4. *Washington Post.* "White House Plans More Oversight of Biotech Foods," *San Francisco Chronicle,* Chronicle Sections, May 3, 2001.
5. *Natural Foods Merchandiser,* "McDonald's Cuts All GMOs in England," August 1999, Website www.healthwellexchange.com/nfm-online/nfm_backs/Aug_99/mcdonalds.cfm.
6. J. Anderson, M.D. and J. Stine. "Detoxing from Toxins." In T. Nichols, M.D., and N. Faass, eds. *Optimal Digestion* (New York: HarperCollins, 1999).
7. E. W. Cutler, *The Food Allergy Cure* (New York: Harmony Books, 2001).
8. N. Cousins, *Anatomy of an Illness* (New York: Bantam, 1991).

CHAPTER ELEVEN

Minimizing Your Exposure to Toxins

Jeffry Anderson, M.D.

For the average American, toxic exposure is subtle and yet ever present. Both low-level and intense exposures can compromise immunity over time and cause a wide variety of symptoms throughout the body. To avoid ongoing exposure, you'll need to think about the source of your drinking water, the safety of your food, and the chemicals in the everyday products you use. One of the most basic approaches involves taking a lifestyle inventory to identify and reduce the chemical burden on your body and your immunity. Remember that some people tend to be more sensitive to toxins than others.

Possible Effects of Toxic Exposure

It is important to lighten any toxic burden that could impair immune function. Symptoms that have been linked to toxic exposure include fatigue, weakness, weight loss, headache, joint and muscle pain, fibromyalgia, and allergic responses. When immune function is compromised, repeated infections can result, such as frequent colds, coughs, flu, bronchitis, or sinus infections. Immune disorders can range from allergic responses to autoimmune diseases such as multiple sclerosis (MS) and Lou Gherig's disease.

- *Damage to immune structures.* Certain toxins can damage fragile immune structures, interfering with the body's ability to produce antibodies. Toxins can also damage white blood cells, including macrophages (scavenger cells), T cells, lymphocytes, and other components of our cellular defenses.
- *Overstimulation of the immune response.* Heavy metals such as cadmium, nickel, and other toxins can increase reactivity, in a chain reaction that can trigger sensitivity to foods, molds, or bacteria. This process can also cause autoimmune conditions to develop, such as lupus or rheumatoid arthritis.

Susan had a five-year history of chronic illness that sometimes became overwhelming. She experienced repeated colds, asthma attacks, and other infections; severe fatigue and joint pain; and difficulty with concentration and memory. Routine medical evaluations found nothing abnormal, and Susan was told she was depressed.

An environmental medicine consultation revealed some significant aspects of her history, including a long-standing hobby of silk-screen printing that involved the use of numerous solvents. Her responses to the questionnaire also indicated that she had dental fillings of mercury-silver amalgam, present since adolescence. Lab tests revealed a number of significant abnormalities. Blood tests showed high levels of toxic solvents: N-hexane, pentane, toluene, and benzene, all used in her silk screening. A urine analysis indicated abnormally high levels of mercury. Additional tests also demonstrated an autoimmune condition involving the thyroid gland and allergic reactions to a number of foods.

After three years of intensive treatment, Susan is finally recovering. To minimize her exposure to heavy metals, she has changed hobbies to avoid using solvents. She also had her mercury fillings replaced by a dentist with special expertise who performed the work over a period of months, taking great care not to reintroduce the mercury back into her body. Once her fillings were removed, her doctor prescribed sauna detox therapy and mercury chelation. She has experienced major improvement in most of her symptoms, in her ability to function, and the quality of her life.

Finding the Cause

Substances in our environment or our food have the potential to be toxic to the body. Toxins — such as industrial chemicals, pesticides, or heavy metals — place a form of stress on the system that can cause imbalances in the body, which may become more severe over time and could result in disease. If damage from toxic exposure occurs to the immune system, the body becomes more vulnerable.

External stressors include:

- Inhalants such as dusts, molds, pollens, and dander
- Chemicals and heavy metals, both synthetic and natural
- Allegernic foods and food additives
- Physical factors such as radiation and electromagnetic fields
- Vibrations, noise, and other stressors

Traces of chemicals such as pesticides can accumulate in the body over time. Thousands of studies have shown the damaging effects of major direct toxic exposure, less research has been done on the effects of long-term exposure to minute doses of toxins. As a result, no one is really sure of the accumulated effects of these chemicals. We do know that cancer rates have doubled in just twenty years and that, unfortunately, childhood cancers have tripled.

At least nine studies have noted an increase in cancers among children whose parents were exposed to pesticides in the workplace. Nineteen other studies found links between pesticide use and childhood cancers. Children living in homes where home and garden pesticides were used were at least twice as likely to develop cancer.

A single intense exposure can cause symptoms as a result of a toxic spill or industrial accident. We know about the effects on people exposed to toxins on the farm or in the workplace from more than a thousand studies in occupational medicine. We also know about the effects on people who live where toxic spills have occurred. Researchers and physicians suggest that these chemicals can cause allergies, chronic fatigue, or even cancer. The effect of any exposure on a person's health depends on their genetic makeup, how well they take care of themselves, and how good their overall health is, as well as their general stress level, and their age.

No one knows the effects of exposure to traces of these chemicals — particularly in combination. We have very few studies, for example, on the interactive effects of food additives. What happens when you eat a hot dog (with nitrates), add mustard and relish (with dyes and sodium benzoate), and drink a diet soda (with aspartame)?

Additional Effects

When immunity is compromised, without the protection of the immune system, the body may become more vulnerable to infection. The drastic effects of lowered immunity are evident, for example, in AIDS conditions.

- *Activation of dormant viruses such as measles and herpes.* When immune integrity is compromised, viruses and other microbes can flourish more easily. Chemical damage can result in the activation of viruses such as measles or herpes, dormant in the body, which can then replicate and spread. This may lead to localized inflammation or to infection anywhere in the body. British research has linked this type of condition, for example, to chronic colitis.

• *Destruction of beneficial microflora.* Damage can also occur to the beneficial flora of the digestive tract, which are often more vulnerable to toxins than harmful bacteria. The good flora produce enzymes and natural antibiotics that can inhibit the invasion of unfriendly microbes. Beneficial flora also synthesize and process nutrients, essential fatty acids, and key vitamins such as B_{12}. In the absence of friendly flora, an overgrowth of harmful microbes can take place. In contrast, research has found that AIDS patients with good flora tend to be healthier.

• *Antibiotic-resistant bacteria.* Mercury (such as that released from dental fillings) can encourage the development of bacteria resistant to antibiotics, including varieties of streptococcus, as confirmed by research. As it turns out, resistance to mercury and antibiotics are both encoded on the bacteria's DNA. This resistance can also be passed on to other bacteria of the same or other species.

Useful Terms

Total load. The total burden of all the stressors at any given time is described as the "total load." Environmental illness may result when the total load becomes too great and the stressors overwhelm the immune system or the cells' defenses.

Adaptability. Our ability to cope with environmental stress and not become ill is also the result of how adaptable we are. The resources that affect our capacity to withstand illness range from our genetic makeup to our economic status. (Research shows that people with low incomes get sick more often than those with high incomes.)

> *Susceptibility.* Our vulnerability to illness is also deter-
> mined by our body's chemistry. Our natural biochemistry
> changes from minute to minute and hour to hour. For
> example, imagine how you feel before you've had a cup of
> coffee — and after. Or how you feel when you're hungry
> and have low blood sugar. What you experience at those
> times are the changes in your body's chemistry.
>
> *Biochemical individuality.* Your inherited body chem-
> istry is unique to your body to some degree. Body chemistry
> may mean we're more susceptible to infection, to addic-
> tions, or to low blood sugar. Other factors include our
> health habits as well as stress and how well we manage it.

Cutting Your Exposure to Toxins

Whether you want to prevent future problems, cut your current
exposure, or detect a problem that may be affecting your health
right now, here's a checklist that you can use to discover problems in
your environment. If any of these factors seem to be an issue for
you, we encourage you to read more about the subject. At the end
of the book in the Resources, you'll find a list of books that explore
this subject in greater depth. Phone numbers and Web addresses for
organizations that provide resources to the public are also included.

- Toxins in water
- Pesticides
- Toxins in the home and garden
- Everyday sources of toxins
- Mercury in dental fillings
- Sick-building syndrome
- Occupational exposures

Toxins in Water

Sources of Exposure

Water is vital to our health, yet it can also be a major source of
chemical exposure. (See chapter 4 for more about water.) Water

often contains fluoride (added for the prevention of cavities) and chlorine. Government testing has also found that it may contain by-products of chlorine interaction (THMs); pesticides, herbicides, and in-organic fertilizer chemicals (such as nitrates); heavy metals (including lead and mercury); petrochemical derivatives, PCBs, and dioxins; and radioactive compounds, such as radium, radon, and uranium, as well as organic matter and bacteria from sewage waste. These findings are based on reviews of federal testing, reported by organizations such as the Environmental Working Group.

Solution

Solving the problem of water additives is a complex subject. One good solution is drinking bottled mountain spring water tested for purity, which is rich in trace mineral content (water stored in glass avoids plastic contaminants). Ask the supplier to send you a copy of the results on their water testing. Installing a water filter or filtration system is another good solution. You'll probably want to do some reading and talk with more than one vendor before you make a purchase. If you have specific requirements or well water, have your water tested before you select the filter. Each system offers benefits and has drawbacks. Reverse-osmosis filters (RO) remove more contaminants from the water than any other system but also remove minerals. Ceramic and carbon-block filters are both respected as generally effective filters.

Pesticides

Sources of Exposure

The United States uses a fifth of the world's pesticides — more than 4.5 billion pounds a year, all sources totaled. Specific pesticide applications in the United States have averaged from 1.2 to 1.5 billion pounds annually for the past twenty years. In developing nations, many pesticides banned here and in Europe are in common use. Worldwide, use of specific pesticides is 6 billion pounds every year.

About half our produce and a third of our grains are reported by the F.D.A. to have pesticide residues. However, by their own report, 90 percent of wheat samples tested contain residues. And the Environmental Working Group found that illegal pesticide levels on imported produce tended to be about twice as high as those reported — averaging 7 percent on some but contaminating as much as 50 percent of the crop in other cases (in 1992 to 1993 federal records). In meat, dairy products, and poultry, testing has found traces of pesticides, hormones, antibiotics, tranquilizers, steroids, or other drugs. In fish and shellfish, possible contaminants include mercury, lead, arsenic, cadmium, chromium, chemicals such as dioxins, and PCBs.

Least Expensive Solutions

You can reduce the residues on some vegetables by peeling. Be sure to buy produce in season as much as possible, since imported produce tends to have higher levels of residues and more illegal pesticides (some countries have less strict pesticide laws). Certain fruits and vegetables test consistently low in residues, while others, such as strawberries and bell peppers, frequently test high, sometimes because of the way they are grown or stored. Minimized your purchase of these, or better yet, only buy them if they're organic. If you can only buy some organic food, you may wish to carry a list in your wallet of the best choices (see the table below).

Most Thorough Solutions

If you have access to certified organic produce and products, buying only or mostly organic food is definitely the best option. You'll taste the difference and you may even notice a difference in your health. This is because truly organic products are not only free of pesticide residues, but they are also raised in soil that is richer in nutrients. Testing has shown increased nutrients in organically raised vegetables from 50 percent to 200 percent. Although organics tend to be a little more expensive, you may come out ahead because of reduced health care costs.

When Organic Food Isn't Available

Strategy	Specifics
Wash vegetables thoroughly	Vegetable washes (usually with a coconut oil base) appear to be helpful; dish detergent gets mixed reviews as a vegetable wash.
Peel vegetables	You can reduce residues on the skin or outer leaves of fruits and vegetables by peeling them. Examples include apples, bananas, grapefruit, oranges, and pears and vegetables such as lettuce, and cucumbers. Corn may still contain residues.
Buy in season	Imported vegetables tend to have higher residues and more toxins, since some chemicals allowed in other countries are more highly toxic.
Avoid foods that test very high for residues of known or illegal toxins	Fruits high in residues include strawberries, peaches and other stone fruits, grapes; vegetables high in residues include celery, bell peppers, green beans, and leafy greens; staples include wheat (tests showed that 90 percent had residues) and rice.
Avoid produce frequently treated with systemic toxins	When systemic toxins are absorbed by produce, they can't be washed off; toxins in animal products are systemic by nature. Buy organics or check a shopper's guide for best choices.
Know the source of the seafood you buy	Buy your seafood from a source you trust; keep up with current information to see what's safe.
Shop wisely	Buy grains in bulk; support your local cooperatives and buying clubs.
Shop selectively	Buy the most important foods organic: baby food, dairy products, meats, and staple grains such as rice and wheat.

Source: T. Nichols, M.D., and N. Faass. *Optimal Digestion.* New York: HarperCollins, 1999. Copyright © Nancy Faass, 1999.

Toxins in the Home and Garden

Sources of Exposure

The main sources of exposure to toxins in the home are solvents such as turpentine, paint and paint thinner, paint and wax strippers, spot removers, degreasers, and gasoline. The most common pesticides found in home and garden are bug sprays, pet sprays, flea collars, and pest strips. These have been consistently linked to higher rates of cancer.

Solutions

You may need to change the products you use, shifting to organic gardening methods and using nontoxic solutions in house cleaning. A number of excellent resources are available. Some offer simple, nontoxic alternatives to household cleaning products. Others provide solutions to complex problems, such as building materials or furnishings. Mail-order catalogs can be useful in purchasing specialty products. (See the Resources.)

You might need to reframe your expectations. If you and your family want to be safe from toxic exposure, you may not be able to have an effortless, picture-perfect lawn with no crab grass. On the other hand, consider the creative possibilities: Minimizing the use of toxins on your lawn may mean planting hardy weed-resistant species of grass or going for a more natural look by putting in a rock garden or planting part of your yard in wildflowers or ivy. You can also have a wonderful garden using the clever techniques of integrated pest management. These strategies minimize the use of toxins and also nurture the land and the environment. Plant flowers and crops that repel pests. Develop healthy soil, mulch for weeds, alternate your crops (intercropping) and rotate them, water your garden deeply and frequently, and encourage natural predators (create a ladybug farm, for example).

Toxins in Household Products

Sources of Exposure

Many familiar products contain additives that can be harmful to the immune system, including fluoride (found in most toothpastes) as well as other toothpaste additives such as propylene glycol (a major constituent of antifreeze), sodium lauryl sulfate, and DEA (di-ethanol-amine). People who are highly sensitive will find that inhaling substances from fabric softeners, colognes, and even scented laundry detergents may make their symptoms worse. Some familiar products are actually quite toxic: For example, lindane is still widely used as a treatment by prescription for lice in children, despite its known neurotoxicity and bioaccumulation.

Solutions

Become informed about which additives are toxic, and then read labels avidly. Consider shifting to simpler products — those without coloring, scents, or complex chemicals. Most health food stores carry a line of safe, nontoxic toothpastes, shampoos, deodorants, and cosmetics. However, it is important to read labels even in health food stores, because some products, such as certain brands of natural toothpaste, now contain fluoride. When you read the cautions on toothpaste labels, you'll notice that the toothpaste manufacturers label fluoride as a toxin and caution that children not be allowed to swallow it. Since these products are widely in use, a realistic goal is not total avoidance but minimizing exposure.

Nontoxic Household Cleaners		
Product	Specifics	Best Option
Dishwashing liquid	May have dye, chlorine, and artificial fragrance	Green products
Dishwasher detergent	Chlorine	Green products are now on the market. Seventh Generation products also available through mail order.
Cleanser	Chlorine; possible asbestos in cleanser	Nonchlorinated scouring powder; available in supermarkets and health food stores; baking soda, borax, salt
Germ-killing disinfectants	Phenol, ethanol, formaldehyde, ammonia, chlorine	$\frac{1}{2}$ cup borax in 1 gallon hot water; aqueous solution of benzalkonium chloride; hydrogen peroxide; "Power Herbal Disinfectant"
Drain cleaners	Lye (poisonous)	1 handful baking soda and $\frac{1}{2}$ cup white vinegar or $\frac{1}{2}$ cup each salt and baking soda followed by hot water; follow by using plunger
Ammonia and all-purpose cleaners	Ammonia (skin irritant, chemical burns); aerosol sprays	1 quart hot water in a spray bottle or bucket with either liquid soap or borax; or green products

	Nontoxic Household Cleaners (continued)	
Product	Specifics	Best Option
Cleaners for appliances	Toxic chemical cleaning agents	$\frac{1}{2}$ tsp. baking soda, 2 tsp. liquid soap, and 2 cups hot water
Oven cleaner	Lye, ammonia, aerosols	Use chemicals carefully for very dirty ovens, or in a spray bottle, 2 Tbsp. liquid soap, 2 tsp. borax, warm water; or make a paste of liquid soap and borax
Glass cleaners	Ammonia, blue dye, aerosol	Solution of $\frac{1}{2}$ water and $\frac{1}{2}$ vinegar in spray bottle or bucket
Mold and mildew cleaners	Kerosene, formaldehyde, phenol, pentachlorophenol	Borax or vinegar and water; dry out the room with heat or a dehumidifier

Source: courtesy of E. Haas, M.D. *The Staying Healthy Shopper's Guide.* Berkeley, Calif.: Celestial Arts, 1999.

Mercury in Dental Fillings

Sources of Exposure

Mercury, silver, and tin are often found in dental fillings (mercury-silver amalgams). These metals may promote antibiotic-resistant gut bacteria and contribute to harmful overgrowth (dysbiois) by species such as klebsiella, citrobacter, and proteus. Mercury is released from dental fillings continuously in very small amounts but can accumulate in the body at dangerous levels.

Mercury-silver amalgams have been outlawed in Europe and Scandinavia for several decades.

People with long-standing multiple mercury-silver fillings may experience generalized problems associated with chronic low-level toxicity from mercury and tin (frequently another component of fillings). Typical symptoms include problems with the nervous or immune system, metabolic disorders, or GI dysfunction.

Solutions

Consider having mercury-silver fillings removed and replaced if possible. It is important to have this procedure performed by a dentist with special training. To remove the fillings, special techniques are used to avoid the reintroduction of mercury into the body, which could cause toxicity and symptoms.

Referrals:

- Foundation for Toxic-Free Dentistry, P. O. Box 608010, Orlando, FL 32860
- Environmental Dental Association (800) 388-8124; for book orders, call the E.D.A. at (619) 586-7626. To receive a list of alternative dentists, send a self-addressed stamped envelope with fifty-five cents' postage. Mail to the E.D.A., P. O. Box 2184, Rancho Santa Fe, CA 92067. Enclose three dollars.

Sick-Building Syndrome

Sources of Exposure

Occupational exposures are frequent or long term, such as one might experience on the job in environments with a high level of synthetic materials including certain paints, some types of synthetic carpets and underpadding, adhesives, formaldehyde, sealers, waxes, disinfectants, cleaning agents, photocopier solution and toner, pesticide applications, and PCBs (from older electrical equipment or fluorescent light transformers). These exposures are worse in tightly insulated buildings that lack adequate ventilation and outdoor air exchange.

Sick-building syndrome can also occur in the home. For example, the pesticide of choice for termite control was traditionally chlordane (an organochloride) until it was banned because of its extreme toxicity. Many homes were treated with chlordane for decades, from the 1950s through the 1970s. It was often injected into the soil under the house. Like DDT, it persists, and since it has a half-life of centuries, it continues to be released. Chlordane causes low-level chlordane toxicity, contaminating the breathable air inside the treated house. If you live in a house built before 1980, check any records on termite treatment.

Solutions

Environmental testing can be obtained for some of the potential toxins and allergens in the home. This may include testing indoor air for formaldehyde and other toxins outgassed from various materials such as sheet rock, particleboard, insulation, and synthetic carpeting. Chlordane used in termite control can be traced through records from the exterminator. Chlordane and radon can also be detected by testing the soil under the house.

Occupational Exposures

Sources of Exposure

Chemical exposures. These concerns are most often associated with the use of chemicals on the job, such as pesticides (agriculture, pest control, and landscaping); solvents (building trades); PCBs, dioxins, and thousands of other chemicals (heavy industry, chemical manufacturing); and petroleum and its by-products (the petrochemical industry). Painters, artists, electricians, gas station attendants, and landscapers may suffer from exposure to solvents.

Heavy-metal exposure. To identify this issue, it is essential that the doctor do a thorough history to look for exposure to heavy metals such as mercury, lead, cadmium, chromium, nickel, tin, or arsenic. Exposures can occur from many sources: 1) devices or materials placed in the body — again, mercury-silver dental amalgams and remnants of orthopedic surgical procedures (stainless steel screws, pins, plates, nails, and wires made of nickel) can be a major source of metal toxicity; 2) residential and commercial sources include paints (particularly lead-based paint or masonry paints, which may contain mercury or thallium), rodenticides, fungicides, pesticides (those containing mercury, arsenic, thallium), and old plumbing with brass fittings or soldered lead joints; and 3) industrial, occupational, or hobby exposures include soldering, welding, foundry work, jewelry making, and artist's materials, especially paints (which contain metals such as cadmium); as well as exposures in numerous industries.

Pesticide exposure. Because of the extremely wide use of many types of pesticides, they are almost impossible to avoid (they include insecticides, fungicides, herbicides, rodenticides, agricultural fumigants, and structural fumigants or wood preservatives). Although pesticides are composed of a wide range of chemical types and molecular structures, almost all have adverse effects on human tissues and organs. Many classes of these chemicals are designed to be toxic to the nervous systems of insects and are toxic to the human nervous system as well. They can also cause problems to the digestive and respiratory systems. Many of these chemicals are clearly toxic to the immune system and bone marrow, and many are associated with the development of cancer.

Solutions

Detoxification is frequently a component of treatment. It should be carried out under medical supervision. Physicians who practice environmental medicine use very specific detoxification techniques, such as oral or IV medication and prescribed nutrients. Although much of detoxification is a natural process, whenever there has been toxic exposure, all treatment should be done under the guidance of a doctor. When chemicals are released during detoxification, it is important that they not recirculate through the body and cause additional damage.

Toxic Exposure and Environmental Medicine

Environmental medicine is considered one of the better approaches to treating the conditions that can result from toxic exposure. Physicians and osteopaths are often the most appropriate practitioners in this field, because they have the legal authority to carry out all aspects of treatment, which may involve ordering medical testing and prescribing medications. When there has been an intensive toxic exposure, it becomes vital that the practitioner have training in toxicology and chelation (clearing the body of metals). The detoxification process releases toxins back into the body, so again, it is extremely important that the toxins not be allowed to recirculate or cause additional damage.

Environmental medicine is considered appropriate therapy in cases of chemical exposure, if symptoms are known to result from exposure to chemicals, heavy metals, or other toxins. It is also an excellent treatment for certain complex illnesses when a condition is long-standing and has not responded to medication or treatment or if there are several symptoms that seem to fluctuate over time. Certain types of illness are linked to toxic exposure, such as sensitivity to chemicals and foods (often called environmental illness), chronic fatigue, or other types of allergies or sensitivities.

Toxic exposure can cause a wide range of physical and neurological disorders including:

- Allergies, sensitivities, and autoimmune conditions: chronic fatigue and environmental illness
- Respiratory disorders: asthma, chronic bronchitis, ear and sinus infections, and frequent sore throats
- Impaired mental functioning: attention deficit disorder, migraine headaches, muscle spasm headaches

- Skin conditions: eczema, dermatitis, and skin discoloration
- Rheumatoid arthritis, fibromyalgia, myalgia, and arthralgia
- Reproductive health issues: fibrocystic breast disease and premenstrual syndrome
- Digestive disorders, including colitis in adults and children

A case history that addresses toxic exposure will alert the physician to a possible environmental component. More serious conditions associated with toxic exposure include heart disease, such as arrhythmias, hypertension, edema, and fluid retention, angina, and myocardial infarction; cancer anywhere in the body; blood disorders, including certain types of anemia; genitourinary conditions: chronic bladder infections, enuresis, recurrent vaginitis, and certain types of infertility; disorders of the nervous system: sleep disorders, certain types of seizures, multiple sclerosis, Parkinson's disease, Alzheimer's disease, and other types of memory problems; behavioral and psychiatric conditions, including irritability, anxiety, eating disorders, sexual dysfunction, panic disorders, manic-depressive illness, and schizophrenia.

Treatment

All therapy, both in the short and long term, must be customized for each client, and may consist of any combination of the following therapies:

- Patient education on the nature of the illness, its treatment, and prevention is a vital part of treatment.
- A therapeutic diet can be customized to the needs of the individual. A diet to reverse deficiencies or to address specific problems may be prescribed by the doctor. These problems could include reactions to food additives, allergies, or other concerns. The doctor may also suggest or prescribe diet and supplements to support healing.

- Supplements can correct or support the body's function. Vital nutrients such as vitamins, minerals, amino acids, and fatty acids may be prescribed to encourage cleansing (detoxification), help heal inflammation or infection (anti-inflammatories), and guard against the effects of toxins (the antioxidants such as A, C, E, and zinc).
- Therapy for the immune system may include customized vaccines made up of specific inhalants, foods, chemicals, or other substances that cause sensitivities. These substances are typically given in tiny doses under the skin (subcutaneous injection) or as tablets taken under the tongue (sublingually).
- Counseling can promote optimal functioning — mentally, emotionally, spiritually, and socially.
- Cleansing (detoxifying therapies) includes a combination of sauna, massage, and exercise designed to clear the tissues of pesticides, chemicals, heavy metals, and other toxins.
- Environmental controls are our efforts to assure that we have clean water and food. They include improving home air quality by minimizing sources of dust, mold, chemicals, and other problems that might be fairly easily to eliminate.
- Doctors may prescribe medications as needed to provide relief from symptoms, while seeking the underlying causes of the problem so they can be corrected. Since patients are already challenged by a toxic burden in the body, any medications should be used strategically in low doses to avoid drug reactions.

Doctors specializing in environmental medicine provide integrative treatment that includes alternative therapies such as detoxification and nutrition. Health issues resulting from toxic exposure require treatment by a practitioner with a broad range of training, who is highly skilled at evaluation.

☞

Jeffry Anderson, M.D., is a physician in environmental medicine. His practice has included the treatment of hundreds of patients who have had environmental exposures, and he has served as consultant on a number of major environmental spills. He received his medical degree from Indiana University, following study at Purdue. He has also specialized in allergy-immunology and applied medical nutrition, using an integral approach to the diagnosis and treatment of chronic disease. Dr. Anderson has provided medical care in a variety of hospital and clinical settings and practiced environmental medicine in Marin County, California, for twenty years until establishing his current consulting practice.

Notes

The American Academy of Environmental Medicine (AAEM). *What Is Environmental Medicine?* (Witchita, KS: AAEM, 1999).

N. A. Ashford and C. S Miller, *Chemical Exposures: Low Levels and High Stakes* (New York: Van Nostrand Reinhold, 1997).

Biological Markers in Immunotoxicology, Multiple Chemical Sensitivities. Addendum to previous title — Environmental Neurotoxicology. Board on Environmental Studies and Toxicology, Commission on Life Sciences, National Research Council (Washington, DC: National Academy Press, 1992).

Doull, Klaassen, Amdur, Eds. *Casarett and Doull's Toxicology, the Basic Science of Poisons* (New York: Macmillan, 1997).

M. Moses, *Designer Poisons.* San Francisco: Pesticide Education Center, 1995.

T. Randolph, *Human Ecology and Susceptibility to the Chemical Environment* (Springfield, IL: Charles C. Thomas Publishers, 1976).

W. Rea, *Chemical Sensitivities.* Vols 1–4 (Boca Raton, FL: Lewis Publishers, 1997).

Department of Adult and Geriatric Health, School of Nursing, University of North Carolina at Chapel Hill, Chapel Hill, NC 27599.

body, mind, and spirit

Dealing with Stress

Jerry Stine, N.C.

Imagine Health

Martin L. Rossman, M.D.

The Role of Spirit in Healing

Len Saputo, M.D.

Piecing the Puzzle Together

Len Saputo, M.D.,
and Nancy Faass, M.S.W., M.P.H.

CHAPTER TWELVE

Dealing with Stress

Jerry Stine, N.C.

Jennie could sense that something was wrong. She frequently had insomnia and never seemed to have any energy, whether or not she slept through the night. She was often irritable or edgy. Every winter she cycled through colds, flu, and sinus infections that required frequent courses of antibiotics, which usually resulted in yeast infections. There seemed to be an association between her frequent illnesses and the long, hectic hours she worked and the fact that she often skipped lunch.

When Jennie went in for a checkup, the exam and blood work turned out to be normal. There was no clear-cut pattern that suggested either a diagnosis or treatment. At that point, she decided to see a nutritionist, one who described his approach as functional nutrition, which evaluates the function of systems such as the liver, digestion, adrenal, and thyroid. Functional nutrition includes the use of diet, vitamin supplements, lifestyle changes, and sometimes referral to medication. The goal is to improve the function of whatever system is out of balance.

Her nutritionist explained that stress is simply the result of any change in our environment that forces us to make an adaptation. Each one of these events causes our body to alter its chemistry — which consumes extra energy and nutrients. This process ultimately has an impact on the adrenal glands, brain chemistry, and the immune system.

Since stress seemed to be a recurring theme in Jennie's life, lab tests were done to check the function of her adrenal glands. The nutritionist explained that the adrenals provide the first response whenever there is stress. These glands can become compromised if the stress continues for an extended period of time. Adrenal stress hormone levels can now easily be measured in saliva through lab testing. Jennie used a home test kit to take samples of her saliva over the course of one day. Then she dropped the kit in the mailbox to the lab.

The results that came back in a few weeks indicated that her adrenal glands were not functioning properly. The pattern of stress hormone output showed extreme highs and lows that were not in sync with her normal chemistry. This pattern indicated that her adrenals were in a constant state of emergency. As a result, Jennie bounced between states of jittery high energy and exhaustion. These elevated levels of stress hormone could also account for her poor sleep.

One of the keys to normalizing adrenal function is to cut down on stress. The nutritionist suggested changes in Jennie's diet and lifestyle that would decrease the wear and tear on her system. She reduced her intake of sweets and starches. She also began working shorter hours and took a yoga class two evenings a week. During the next three months, these simple changes brought real progress.

Her energy returned. She found that her sense of edginess was gone and that she was seldom sick.

Looking back, she realized that the stress involved more than just the emotional factors in her life — like worrying about a deadline or disagreeing with her boss. It was the total of all the demands she placed on her body and mind, including working long hours under pressure, skipping meals, binge eating, losing sleep, and everything else. Fortunately, she was able to change these patterns before they caused more serious problems.

Too much stress can overwork or disrupt the body's hormone output. Stress also affects immunity indirectly, with an impact on the levels of T cells and antibodies. Both high and low adrenal function can result in symptoms anywhere in the body.

The Effects of Stress

Common Symptoms	Health Conditions
• Frequent illness	• Immune suppression
• Slow healing	• Autoimmune conditions such as lupus
• Inflammation	• Thyroid disorders
• Joint pain or tendonitis	• PMS and other symptoms in younger women
• Insomnia	• Menopause syndrome in midlife women
• Recurring fatigue	• A variety of symptoms affecting midlife men
• Difficulty with mental tasks	• Loss of sexual interest or function
• Difficulty coping emotionally	• Accelerated aging
	• Osteoporosis
	• Arthritis
	• A variety of digestive disorders
	• Increased cancer risk

The Effects of Stress on Immunity

There are important links between stress, hormones, and immunity. Our basic understanding of how this occurs was mapped out by Hans Selye in his groundbreaking research on stress in the 1930s.[1] Seyle studied animals placed under stress for long periods of time and found that their production of adrenal hormones was seriously compromised. As a result, important aspect of immune function actually began to deteriorate. Selye observed that the effects of stress are so powerful that they eventually shut down major immune defenses. He observed that long-term stress caused the adrenal glands to wither, deterioration of the thymus gland (where T cells are made), atrophy of lymph tissue (the source of most of our protective antibodies), and the development of ulcers.

- *Stress can decrease T cell production.* Under long-term stress, the thymus gland begins to shrivel and atrophy. Drops in T cell production occur in connection with stress — even short-term stress — and have been confirmed in study after study in both animals and humans.
- *Stress can lower antibody levels.* There is a link between adrenal signals and antibody production. When the adrenals are affected by stress, antibody output is also affected, whether the adrenals are under- or overproducing stress hormones. The majority of the body's immunity and antibody production is located in the digestive tract. Selye's research also observed atrophy in the lining and lymph tissue of the digestive tract where the antibodies are made. This loss leaves the system extremely vulnerable to infection from bacteria present in food or water. This also creates the potential for candida overgrowth.

Extended stress can compromise the majority of our immune defenses. However, we can't use symptoms alone as an indication of what's going on in the body or with the adrenals. Nor do symptoms alone provide an indication of what kind of treatment is required. Adrenal function and adrenal output (cortisol levels) must also be tested.

Stress and Lifestyle

We can become better skilled at recognizing the causes of stress in our own lives as they occur — whether they're physical, emotional, or lifestyle factors. We'll describe typical treatment of stress-related symptoms later in this chapter. First, let's take a closer look at how stress is evaluated.

Assessing Stress

When psychologists assess the level of stress in a patient's life, they begin by evaluating lifestyle factors. They use a checklist that identifies intense life events likely to cause stress — for example, being in an accident, having surgery, losing a job, or getting divorced. Stress can also result from pleasant but disruptive events such as getting married, traveling, or getting a new job. Even intense joy is a form of stress on the body. The key to stress is not whether it is pleasant or unpleasant but whether it makes continuous demands on our body's deep reservoirs of vitality.

Long-term stress can have a profound impact on the mind and body. For example, having a number of children in close succession is stressful because of the physical demands of pregnancy and the exertion of caring for young children. Also, caring for a family member who has an extended illness can be extremely stressful. In an evaluation of stress on a person's life, each event is assigned a score suggesting its intensity. Then the scores of all the stressors are compiled to measure and reflect the level of stress.

In the field of environmental medicine, the sum of all these stressors on an individual is described as the "total load." This implies the accumulated effect of all the stresses on the body and mind. We are accustomed to thinking of highly emotional situations as the main source of stress. But the total burden of stress extends beyond mental and emotional factors and can even include routine daily events such as driving on the freeway during rush hour. In terms of the body and its physiology, stress includes the challenge of infection, injury, chemical exposure, or medical procedures. Intense physical events from running a marathon to having a baby are also stressors. Sources of stress also include factors in our body chemistry, such as waiting too long to eat (resulting in low blood sugar) or having frequent reactions from food allergies.

Stress and the Body

Humans and animals have similar basic reactions to stress — the "flight or fight response." When confronted by danger or challenges, adrenal hormones begin coursing through our bloodstream to prepare us for action: to fight or to make a rapid retreat. Although we commonly refer to this experience as an "adrenaline" rush, the hormone actually triggered by stress is cortisol. Cortisol is produced by the adrenal glands, so it's logical that cortisol levels provide important clues to understanding the effects of stress on the body. There are various patterns of stress response.

Pattern One: Overwhelm

Excessive cortisol output — hyperadrenal response — tends to occur in young people who experience frequent stress. Testing and evaluation often provide the basic information we need to return those functions to balance. Problems seem to occur in people who are locked into a lifestyle pattern of stress. Each specific event in a stressful lifestyle, when viewed in isolation, doesn't appear to be a problem. But it is the continuous stress from multiple sources that tends to be the most harmful. Chronic stress creates a situation in which the adrenal function is basically *always* in the flight-or-fight position, day and night. This syndrome is described as stress-response maladaption, meaning that the body is not able to shift from the stress response back into normal function. This condition can result from lifestyle issues, diet, food reactions, infection, or the use of certain medications, overwork, intense athletic activity, and mental and emotional strain. The greatest daily source of stress for most people is their diet. The major factors are a diet high in sweets and starches or hidden food allergies. Any high stress, particularly metabolic stress, will affect adrenal function.

Just imagine the effects on your body if it were pumping out high levels of cortisol, day after day. Just as you would suspect, the initial responses resembles a coffee jag: increased nervousness, mood swings, fatigue, food cravings, and chronic insomnia. The long-term effects can include immune suppression, hormone imbalances, premature aging, chronic fatigue, and psychological symptoms and can be experienced anywhere in the body.

Pattern Two: Burnout

Adrenal depletion — low adrenal output — is not rare or unusual. When people overreact or act out on the job or with their family, this behavior often reflects the consequences of chronic stress — the stress syndrome, the result of many years of hyperadrenal response. In our society, we are continually under multiple stressors that can stimulate a hyperadrenal output. Over time, this chronic stress literally wears out the body's ability to maintain a hyperstress response condition. This long-term overstimulation leads to the loss of the body's ability to adapt. It is in midlife that both men and women clearly begin to experience the effects of chronic stress.

In older clients, there is a tendency toward underactive adrenal function. In some people, this can result from a type of adrenal depletion caused by many years of chronic stress and excessive adrenal output. Long-term stress can literally wear out the ability of the adrenals to adapt. The loss of this capacity often reflects years of overstimulation from the same fundamental stressors that we saw in pattern one: stressful lifestyle, overwork, addiction, diet, allergies, or chronic infection. Again, these factors can all contribute to the symptoms of aging.

More Problems with Adrenal Burnout

When the adrenals become depleted, there are two principal consequences. The first is a level of cortisol that is too low to properly regulate other hormone levels, immune response, or brain activity. When the adrenals can't supply adequate levels of cortisol, it becomes more difficult to produce the immediate response that's required in cases of emergency (the cortisol burst). Cortisol not only initiates the stress response, it also has a role in turning it off. In addition, the cortisol burst is important, because it initiates some aspects of immune function and turns off certain inflammatory processes.

Either overactive or underactive adrenals can cause impaired immune function. Laboratory testing is usually necessary to assess the health of the adrenals. The test results indicate the pattern of cortisol output of the client, enabling the health-care practitioner to develop therapy tailored specifically to the client's needs.

Treatment and Testing

We can take many different approaches to treat the conditions that may result from chronic stress.

- *Reduce stress.* The first step is to identify any stress caused by lifestyle and to take steps to eliminate or minimize it. This topic is so vast that it is the central theme of not one book but many. You may want to take a systematic approach to stress, identifying one area at a time and bringing it into balance. Sometimes going back to the basics of sleep and drinking water are good first steps. You may also want to take a look at chapters 5 and 13 respectively for more about healing exercise and mind-body medicine.
- *Use good nutrition.* Another good place to begin is to focus on the diet by reducing stressors such as allergenic foods and by improving nutritional support. Typically, treatment includes:

1. Stabilizing blood sugar
2. Choosing foods that reduce the body's need for insulin
3. Supplementing diet with certain vitamins, minerals, and/or hormones
4. Identifying food allergies or sensitivities

(Also see chapter 8 for more about eating well and stabilizing blood sugar and chapter 9 for more about food allergies.)

Testing

Testing can be another important step in determining your nutritional needs. For the past ten years, a range of useful new lab tests have been developed in an emerging field called functional medicine. This particular type of testing is available through physicians who practice preventive medicine and through some nutritionists. Functional testing is one of the most important components of new approaches to nutrition. The tests provide additional insight into the functioning of various body systems such the adrenals and the liver. Some of these simple, inexpensive tests can be performed in a doctor's office, and others can be done at home.

- *Determining how the body is functioning.* This lab work provides feedback that can help us correct conditions such as the "stress syndrome." The test results indicate how key systems, such as the adrenals, liver, or digestive system, are working. The goal is to gain information that will inform the development of a personalized program in nutrition and lifestyle.
- *Identifying nutritional needs.* In the early years of nutritional therapy, practitioners made most of their recommendations based only on their client's symptoms. There was little testing available beyond lab work such as blood tests for iron deficiencies. Now we have testing that provides more information on nutritional status.

These tests have changed our understanding of how disease develops and of how to intervene before it develops. The testing allows us to better determine what individual clients require and to tailor nutritional programs to their specific needs.

This information provides the basis for recommendations on diet and supplements. With this type of information, we can develop a nutritional program that is not just based on general ideas about nutrition or current trends in the field. Instead, nutritional therapy is based on the client's health status, reflected in the testing. These lab evaluations are taking the guesswork out of the practice of clinical nutrition.

- *Checking the effectiveness of treatment.* By retesting we can assess the effectiveness of our programs objectively. After a client has undergone a course of nutritional therapy, retesting is essential to determine whether the treatment is working and what to do next. By performing the same test at a later time, we can tell if the deficiency or imbalance has been corrected and to what degree. That feedback guides the next stage of the therapy.

Testing for Stress

For clients with stress syndrome, there are two particular tests that are most often used. Practitioners almost always check the status of the adrenals. The other test is for food allergies.

Adrenal testing. We are now able to evaluate some aspects of adrenal function using simple inexpensive saliva tests. Through this information, we assess the wear and tear on the body and on the adrenals glands. By evaluating the client's lab work, diet, health history and by factoring in age and gender, we are able to identify adrenal patterns that may be out of balance and to recommend nutritional therapy.

Allergy testing. Hidden food allergies can be a major form of stress. Yet in most cases, it is very difficult to determine the source of the allergy or sensitivity. Most food allergies tend to have a delayed onset. Often the reactions are due to foods that people consume frequently. Over time, food allergies and sensitivities can cause low-grade irritation and inflammation. Improved tests are now available that can be useful in identifying allergies (through blood, saliva, or skin testing). (Chapter 9 reviews some of the major forms of allergy testing.)

Symptoms Improved by Treating Stress

When we are able to decrease the demands on the body from lifestyle and metabolic stress, a surprising number of symptoms tend to gradually improve.

Stress syndrome. Our ability to respond to stress and then return to normal function (overcoming the stress syndrome) is the essence of the flexibility that determines good health. The minute we are under stress, the adrenal glands begin to react. Until the stress abates — or until our sense of emergency abates — the adrenals are constantly involved in our hormonal adaptation to stress. Being stuck in a high-stress situation over a long period of time can compromise systems throughout the body, such as hormone production. So it is essential to address and correct adrenal stress syndrome to have optimal health.

Coping ability. Nutritional and lifestyle therapy can enhance the ability to cope with stressful situations. With these kinds of therapies, clients experience an improved tolerance for stress, particularly in interactions with others, with less tendency to be reactive or overly emotional. Negative patterns — such as irritation, anger, depression, or withdrawal — begin to subside. Life often becomes less overwhelming.

Insomnia. Long-term stress can lead to insomnia and fatigue. Disturbances in sleep can caused by either an overactive or depressed adrenal function. Since the corrections for these two profiles are quite different, it is important to use testing that will indicate which pattern is present.

Fatigue and low energy. People with fatigue or chronic fatigue syndrome very frequently benefit from these interventions. Energy production seems to parallel the output of the adrenals. In situations where there are energy dips during the day (typically in the afternoon), they tend to parallel a drop in cortisol levels. These fluctuations become apparent in the results from the saliva testing and may be modified through a nutritional program.

Weight gain. Often our appetite is influenced by the chain reactions that result from hormonal influences. For example, adrenal output is known to affect the hypothalamus, a tiny gland in the midbrain that regulates appetite. The hypothalamus also regulates other aspects of metabolism, such as thirst and sleep patterns. So disturbances in adrenal output can indirectly affect appetite, thirst, or sleep. Weight loss is frequently observed as one of the outcomes of an adrenal-balancing program.

The stress syndrome frequently occurs in people who are consuming a diet high in refined starches and sweets (high glycemic foods). This type of diet typically causes weight gain and the risk of obesity. We now know that foods that overtax insulin production are a form of stress on the body. Cravings for carbohydrates can result from any number of causes, including a response to high stress. One way out of this vicious cycle involves eating foods that do not cause the production of too much insulin. The trick is to learn to use the Glycemic Index skillfully. Identify your favorite foods on the Index and use them as the basis for your shopping list and menus. This is not as challenging as it sounds, since many low-glycemic foods are standard favorites. (For more information on this important aspect of stress reduction, see chapter 8.)

Conditions Improved by Treating Stress

A wide range of chronic health issues can also be improved by treating stress.

Inflammatory conditions. Stress treatment can lead to improvements in many types of inflammation, including arthritis and fibromyalgia; allergies, asthma, and chronic sinus infections; dermatitis and a wide range of skin problems; and chronic heartburn, peptic ulcers, colitis, or other conditions related to digestion. In people with inflammatory disorders, immune function may be depressed, delayed, or overstimulated. In these complex situations, therapy is always provided on an individual case-by-case basis. Any intervention should be based on testing, with follow-up evaluations to assure that the therapy is on track. Nutritional interventions for most inflammatory conditions include individualizing the diet, improving digestive function, reducing stress, improving lifestyle, and providing adrenal support.

Arthritis. At one time, arthritis was considered primarily a problem involving the muscles and joints, a purely structural problem. Now evidence points to an immune involvement in arthritic conditions — an autoimmune reaction within the joint that causes pain, inflammation, loss of function, and possible damage. Individuals with arthritis symptoms may be at risk from serious immune system defects, so it is important to address both the arthritis and any abnormalities in immunity. Nutritional therapy and counseling to reduce inflammation from arthritis includes specific supplements to build quality connective tissue and the general strategies mentioned above.

Autoimmune conditions. In these disorders, the immune system is inappropriately attacking the body tissue, resulting in conditions such as certain types of arthritis or lupus. Although many disorders are grouped together under this term, not all of them actually fit the definition of autoimmunity. Almost any condition that includes inflammation has the potential to involve an autoimmune reaction. There is a bewildering array of autoimmune disorders, and many of them respond to the same therapies used to correct stress syndrome.

Migraines. These mysterious and debilitating headaches seem connected to a wide range of metabolic stresses. Fortunately migraines and chronic headaches may also respond to the program used to address stress syndrome.

Hormone imbalances. It is not unusual for clients with stress syndrome also to have hormone imbalances. In younger women, typical symptoms can include premenstrual syndrome, cycle irregularities, decreased sex drive, and premature menopause. In midlife women with stress syndrome, the symptoms of menopause tend to be more severe. In correcting these conditions, it can be effective to address the adrenal imbalance first. Clients often respond just as if we had corrected their hormone situation directly. For that reason, we do not usually do in-depth testing for hormone levels until we have provided a basic nutritional program. In these cases, about two-thirds of the hormone imbalances are self-correcting without any direct intervention.

Thyroid imbalances. Hormone balance frequently presents a complex picture. Thyroid imbalances can be characterized by low body temperature, low energy, and excessive weight loss or gain. Often skin ages prematurely, and hair thins. Some clients report that even prescribed thyroid medication has not cleared up their symptoms. In certain cases, these clients have responded well when adrenal function is brought back into balance through nutritional therapy. This type of issue is an example of how a functional approach can address a series of related symptoms.

Heart problems. When adrenal function is out of balance, the effects of stress on the heart also tend to be greater. Vulnerable plaque is a serious immunological situation that typically occurs because of the effects of long-term stress. For example, it can cause thrombosis, a type of heart attack. Therapies that address stress syndrome, combined with nutritional support for immune function, can reduce the risk of this situation.

Cancer risk. People with low-grade immune dysfunction may be at increased risk of a number of more serious conditions, including cancer. By enhancing basic immunity, we are not only improving health in the short term but also addressing processes that have significant impact on degenerative disease. It is vital to remember this as an important goal when rebuilding immune function. Keeping the immune system intact is one of the best defenses we have in reducing the risk of cancer and other dangerous conditions.

We have seen that as stress persists, overall health begins to decline. The adaptive range of coping response narrows, and the capacity to handle stress is reduced. There is a sense of loss of control — that one is being victimized by the normal events of daily life. Fortunately, that process is almost always reversible with lifestyle and nutritional therapy. People frequently report that their ability to cope with stressful situations becomes quite enhanced. Clients report that they have a greater ability to tolerate stress and an increased sense of wholeness.

ى

Jerry Stine, N.C., is a nutritional consultant and the director of the Lifespan Institute, which he founded in 1987. Lifespan provides individual nutritional consultations by phone and access to a variety of the latest functional testing, including evaluations for allergies, adrenal function, and nutritional status. The Lifespan Institute can be contacted at (415) 479-3552.

Notes

1.   H. Selye, *The Stress of Life,* 2d ed. (New York: McGraw-Hill Professional, 1978).

CHAPTER THIRTEEN

Imagine Health

Martin L. Rossman, M.D.

Alexandra was thirty years old, active and successful, but worried. She had developed a number of lumps in her breast. Several physicians had diagnosed them as benign nodules, but she worried that they were precancerous and wanted to know if she could do anything to make them go away. Alexandra was intensely involved in every aspect of her life. She worked long hours, traveled frequently in her work, and kept a busy social schedule as well. She often felt tense and tired, and she wanted less stress in her life, though she saw that stress as a problem separate from her breast lumps.

As part of our consultation, I asked her to relax and let an image of the lumps come to mind. She imagined them as rocks in a stream and was upset to see they were partially obstructing its flow. As she looked more closely, however, her perception of the rocks changed dramatically. She noticed that they were very smooth, shiny, and lustrous and looked more like pearls than rocks.

Alexandra immediately understood that, like pearls in an oyster, these lumps had formed in response to irritation and represented an attempt to protect her from further harm.

When I asked her what would need to happen for the pearls to dissolve, she sensed a need to "remove the source of irritation." She consequently made changes in her scheduling, her traveling, and her diet, and the lumps in her breast disappeared within a few months.

Our feelings are widely acknowledged to be the essence of what it means to be human. If this is true, it is logical that the mind and emotions have a role in healing, and research bears this out. Although this is widely acknowledged and supported, we tend to overlook the role of mental and emotional factors when we are under stress or when we get sick.

Health and illness in some respects are still a great mystery, despite the tremendous gains made by science and medicine. For example, some people do all the right things, eat all the right foods, take all the right supplements — and yet are sick all the time. Others do all the wrong things, eat all the wrong things, smoke, and take other risks — yet remain healthy. The effects of the mind on the body offer one of the missing pieces in this puzzle. In practical terms, we can use our minds to improve our health and well-being. The effects of the mind and spirit on the body are now being systematically studied in a field described as psychoneuroimmunology. This chapter offers glimpses of this emerging field and practical tools for applying mind-body techniques in your own life.

The Effects of the Mind on Health

The study of mind-body interactions offers new evidence of the important connections between our thought processes and the function of our physiology. They manifest as chain reactions throughout the body. Much of what we now understand about this dynamic was unknown until about ten years ago. For example, our thoughts and emotions affect the hypothalamus, a small gland in the brain that influences many other biochemical systems. The hypothalamus:

- Runs the autonomic nervous system — the "automatic" system that regulates breathing, heartbeat, and other vital functions
- Governs the secretion of neurotransmitters that carry the brains messages to the body
- Affects the production of our hormones
- Influences the production of adrenal hormones that help us cope with stress
- Directly stimulates the thymus and the lymph nodes, the source of T cells and antibodies

These are just a few examples of the innumerable ways in which our thoughts actually influence the workings of the body and its chemistry. The mind-body connection is reflected in every aspect of our lives from our cells to our behavior:

Lifestyle. How we live on a day-to-day basis has a major effect on how healthy we are. To the degree that we choose our lifestyle, our mind and emotions influence our behaviors related to diet, alcohol, drugs, smoking, driving, stress management, coping responses, and even our choice of health care. Our self-image and belief systems are reflected in our answers to questions such as, What do I deserve? How do I make choices? What other options are available to me?

Genetics. In the past, we have viewed other aspects of health as beyond our control. Throughout the twentieth century, our genetic heritage was believed to be unchangeable. We now know, however, that many of our genes are regulatory — that they switch on and off for reasons that have not yet been discovered. Research shows that some of the lifestyle choices we make, such as diet, can affect how these genes are expressed (known as genetic expression).

Mental and emotional influences on immunity may also turn genes on and off.

Response to treatment. How well we comply with our health-care practitioners' recommendations for us is also affected by mindset. Whether the doctor recommends the right nutrients or medication does not matter if the patient doesn't take them. A good treatment for diabetes, for example, doesn't have much value if patients don't comply with it. In general, how a person responds to their illness is a critical factor in the progression of healing.

Immunity. Perhaps the clearest indication of the mind's influence on the body is how powerfully stress-reducing techniques affect our health.[1,2] We know from research that people who engage in regular sessions of relaxation, meditation, or visualization can enhance their T cell responses to cancer or chronic viral illnesses. It's also been shown that these techniques can enhance other aspects of their immune chemistry and the aggressiveness of their T cells. This effect is so significant, that if it were a medication, all doctors would prescribe it. Yet it occurs simply in response to the power of the mind.

Stress reduction. Most of us think of the influence of the mind on the body in terms of stress and intense emotions. We now know that many health issues are associated with the effects of stress, which raises the question of what we can do to counteract these influences. Since the mind is probably the greatest producer of stress, achieving mental composure and inner calm offers a fairly direct way to restore balance. Some of the most effective stress reducers are those that engage and relax the mind, such as relaxation techniques, meditation, biofeedback, hypnosis, and imagery.

The Mind-Body Connection and Imagery

Imagery is an important key to mind-body healing, because it is the code language of the mind, the body, and the spirit. Imagery simply means thinking in the sensory mode — in mental images that engage the senses. It is a very efficient language that can provide access to deeper levels of experience, emotion, and memory. Consider imagery in this context. Have you ever literally worried yourself sick?

- Ever worried until you had a headache?
- Worried until your shoulders grew tense?
- Have you ever been unable to sleep because of worry?

If any of these experiences describe you (as they do most of us), that's a sign that you are already good at imagery. If you stay awake at night imaging things that might happen — and are able to imagine them so vividly that it creates anxiety reactions in your body and your chemistry, you already know how to use imagery. You have established a strong mind-body connection. Since the body is not designed to be in the stress mode constantly, the next step is to learn to use the mind-body connection to send different signals through the same pathways. There is nothing wrong with your mind-body connection — it's just that when you worry you arouse the body in a stress response. You can also learn to send signals that stimulate the relaxation response. In fact, you can learn to call up this response at will. Consider, for example, that when the stress response abates and your body goes into a relaxation response, blood coagulation comes down five or six times. These are real effects that can be used in the management of stress. (What cardiologists would not be interested in a medication that reduced blood clotting at least fivefold?)

Stress and Illness: Taking Back Control

To some degree, all illness is ultimately stress related. Since stress either causes or aggravates illness or the illness itself creates stress, it would be ideal if stress management were always a component of treatment for people with serious conditions.

Yet it can also be said that stress has nothing to do with illness. It is stress *tolerance*, not *stress* itself, that makes the difference. It is not always what happens to you that causes the illness, but how you respond to it — how resilient you are and how well you cope. That is not to deny that catastrophic things happen. But many people seem to be made ill by things that they can't define — worries that nag at them and cause tremendous anxiety and physiological distress. This distress is reflected in a broad range of symptoms:

- Back pain
- Irregular heartbeat
- High blood pressure
- Colitis
- Migraine headaches

Although there are usually specific treatments that can be directed at symptoms, they often bring about improvement but not cure. Unless a shift is made in the way we live, true healing may not occur. Relaxation can be a useful tool in restoring personal balance. Although it's a natural response, for most of us it is one we need to relearn. Imagery is one of the easiest ways to relax, by simply thinking with your senses. An image is a thought that has sensory qualities — a memory, fantasy, or a dream that engages the senses.

When doctors and their clients work together using this format, we call it Interactive Guided Imagery. For example, we use this method to assist clients who have a serious illness that hasn't responded to treatment. As the client describes their inner world and their experience using their senses, they become more and more subjectively engaged with that inner reality. The process requires them to access a great deal of sensory information. This sensory recruitment is the gateway to a number of important benefits, including:

- Access to some of their deepest feelings, to the subconscious, insight into issues that may be eluding them consciously
- Clues to overcoming these issues
- A means to elicit the relaxation response

Relax

Take a few deep breaths, and let your breathing become deeper and more regular...

Notice the fresh air and oxygen you're breathing in as you inhale.

When you exhale, let go and become even more deeply relaxed.

You may also want to go through your body mentally, inviting different areas to relax.

Now imagine going to some place that is very peaceful, safe, and beautiful — some place where you feel good.

It might be a place you've been at some time in your life, or it may be a place that exists only in your imagination — it doesn't matter, as long as it tranquil.

Now, take a look around...

What do you see?

What does it look like in that beautiful, quiet place?

What are the colors?

Define everything in as much detail as you would like, using all five of your senses.

What sounds do you hear... is it very quiet?

What is the weather like today?

What season is it?

What is the temperature?

What time of day does it seem to be?

Find the place where you feel the most comfortable, and enjoy the peacefulness and relaxation you feel there, for as long as you'd like.

When you are ready, slowly and gently let the images fade and bring your attention back to the outer world.

The effects of imagery on the brain are in some ways comparable to the effects of real experience. We know a great deal about the process from MRI research that monitors the brain while subjects are performing imagery. For example, when people imagine hearing music, songs, or voices, the portion of the brain in which they process auditory information becomes active. When they visualize images, the visual centers in the brain are activated. When they imagine walking, the motor area of the brain becomes engaged.

In using imagery, by focusing on information from your senses, your subjective reality becomes real. The body responds by shifting into the relaxation response. And why shouldn't it? It's receiving vivid input from the various centers of the brain, including the auditory, visual, spatial, and motor areas. So just as the body responds to thoughts like, How am I going to make the next mortgage payment? What happens if I lose my job? it also responds to positive images of tranquility.

The most common form of imagery is worry. When we learn to use that same skill in a different way, we have developed a powerful means for accessing our inner reality, solving problems, and engaging the relaxation response.

Ed came to me ten years ago complaining of recurrent sinus infections, constant hay fever, and severe daily headaches above and behind his eyes. Regular doses of aspirin, decongestants, and antihistamines were of minimal help. Conventional allergy testing showed he was sensitive to many pollens and airborne chemicals. He was much worse on smoggy days and when the pollen count was high. Years of allergy shots had helped somewhat but had lost their effectiveness in the year preceding his visit to me. Ed was a busy, caring person, deeply involved with his family, church, and community. He was interested, informed, and concerned about the world. I noticed right away that Ed's brow was deeply furrowed and that he looked worried. He had come to me to see if acupuncture could help him, and we set up a series of appointments for treatments.

We also talked about the possible role of stress in his symptoms, and I suggested that he take home a relaxation tape. The next week he came in for his first acupuncture treatment and happily reported he was "already 90 percent better." He had been enjoying the relaxation and had noticed a major improvement in his symptoms. After a few acupuncture treatments he was free of headaches and allergy symptoms. He has continued to use the relaxation technique regularly and in ten years has had no sinus infections or severe headaches and needs no medications. He comes for an acupuncture treatment every year or two if the pollution levels are unusually high and he develops symptoms. He feels that learning to relax made a bigger change in his health than anything else he had ever tried.

More Benefits of Imagery

If you have a condition such as arthritis, chronic pain, fibromyalgia, or diabetes, you may want to explore the benefits of imagery. For anyone with health problems, imagery can be a useful adjunct to treatment. It is important to remember that imagery and other mind-body approaches are not intended to replace medical treatment, but they can help manage health and stress and access inner strengths.[3]

A tremendous amount of research suggests that how we think affects the outcome of our treatment.

Consider a study conducted at the University of California, Davis, in which surgical patients were instructed on the use of imagery to minimize blood loss and enhance healing.[4,5] In a five-minute interview the day before surgery, a psychologist prepared patients with the following information. "Have you ever noticed that when you get embarrassed, you blush? That is because your body knows how to shunt blood from one place to another. Your body is so smart, it can also shunt the blood away from the site of surgery (if you suggest that through your mental images). This will minimize blood loss during the procedure. Afterward, it would also be helpful to bring the circulation back to that area, to provide the nutrients and oxygen you need for tissue repair."

These instructions were given for about five minutes. The doctor did not use formal hypnosis, although certainly people are hypersuggestive right before surgery. The results? Blood loss in the group that received mental preparation for surgery averaged 45 percent less (600 cc of blood compared to 1,100 cc of blood lost among people who had not had this five-minute preparatory session).

Practical Applications

The use of imagery in healing and self-healing has very practical applications.

Connecting with your inner strengths. It's amazing how much self-knowledge each of us have. Imagery provides another opportunity to connect with that basic intelligence and to express it. The idea is to relax deeply and get in touch with the part of you that knows the most about healing, which you may envision as your inner healer or inner physician. Ask your physician what is important for you to know and to do. A study on imagery at the chemotherapy unit of University of California, San Francisco, used guided imagery tapes. After just one session with the tapes, patients were able to get relief from anxiety and depression they were feeling. Other studies have shown relief from nausea and vomiting relating to chemotherapy. These patients were better able to tolerate treatment and more likely to finish the course of treatment.

Accessing information from the subconscious and gaining insight into your issues. The idea in this process is to help you access your own capabilities, your own process of imagery, which is actually how we navigate through the world. You may use it to gain insight into elusive symptoms or into those with a psychological component. In either situation, imagery can facilitate a conversation with your body, opening a kind of inner dialogue.

Working through emotional blocks to your self-care. Imagery and mind-body activities expand the ability to become self-aware, to try different behaviors, to learn, and to experiment constructively.

Reducing stress and worry. Imagery can help us cope with anxiety and depression. These are emotions that tend to amplify symptoms when people are under stress or facing situations of uncertainty. Imagery can provide patients with greater control over fear or worry.

Preparing for medical treatment. As we've seen, imagery can be a useful mental tool in preparing for and tolerating treatment or surgery. It can support patients in their decision making, helping to overcome inner barriers such as fear.

More Benefits of the Mind-Body Approach

A tremendous body of research from the past thirty years supports the effectiveness of psychosocial and mind-body interventions, ranging from patient education and support groups to imagery, relaxation, and hypnosis.

Empowerment. The value of patient education was tracked for four hundred people with severe arthritis.[6,7] They were provided with six two-hour sessions that included relaxation, information on how to communicate with their doctor, assertiveness skills, and active coping skills. For the next two years, the Stanford study tracked these patients, and found that they experienced 20 percent less pain and major decreases in depression and anxiety. Although their conditions were as severe as those of nonparticipants, they were much more functional in their lives and had increased sense of self-efficacy. A comparable six-year study of melanoma patients found that those who received coaching and education had 20 percent the mortality of those who did not. They also had improved immunity (measured in T cell levels), better functioning, decreased depression and anxiety, and increased sense of self-efficacy.[8]

Support. One of the major findings over the past decade has been that people in support groups become survivors. A Stanford study of women with advanced metastatic cancer found that those in support groups lived twice as long, on average, as women with comparable conditions who were not in support groups.[9,10]

A way to work collaboratively with a health-care practitioner. These techniques can provide patients with better access to resources they can bring to the physician-client relationship. As a doctor, I know that without my clients' involvement what we can accomplish will be severely limited. On the other hand, if they bring what they know to the healing process, and I bring what I know, we have the best chance of successful healing.

Pain relief. Mind-body techniques are well known as tools for coping with chronic pain.[11] The studies suggest that people experience less pain and discomfort (for example, 50 percent less postoperative discomfort in procedures such as abdominal surgery). As a result, they need less narcotic medication, less care, and tend to have more successful recovery.[12,13,14]

Wellness. Imagery and mind-body methods can aid patients in reshaping their self-image. After a lifetime of chronic illness, it is understandable that some patients cannot imagine themselves as healthy. Assisting them on the road to healing means that they must envision their life in a different way, answering the essential question, What would your life be like if you were healthy?

Precautions and Contraindications

Imagery is a noninvasive method that can provide increased self-control and self-efficacy. That said, it is not for everyone.

Some patients become more anxious when they attempt to relax, which may be due to either physical or psychological factors. Although this anxiety can be worked with, it usually requires the assistance of a professional trained in the use of imagery. This is not an appropriate form of treatment for people with mental illness such as severe psychosis, associative disorders, or borderline personality disorder unless the therapist is well trained in this technique.

It is important to restate that using imagery is not a replacement for appropriate treatment. It is also not an implication of guilt. Just because you can help yourself with your mind doesn't mean that you created your illness or that you are flawed because you are ill. Actually, learning to use your imagination skillfully is an active role you can take to help yourself achieve the best possible state of health.

$$\approx$$

Martin Rossman, M.D., is founder and director of the Collaborative Medicine Center. He is codeveloper of Interactive Guided Imagery, and cofounder of the Academy for Guided Imagery and the Imagination Foundation. Trained at the University of Michigan, he is a faculty associate at the University of California, San Francisco, the California School of Professional Psychology, and John F. Kennedy University. Dr. Rossman is active as board member of the Stanford Corporate Health Project and the Rosenthal Center for Complementary Medicine in New York. He is the author of *Guided Imagery for Self-Healing.* Dr. Rossman can be reached for consultations in Mill Valley, California, at (415) 363-3197. The Academy for Guided Imagery can be contacted at (800) 726-2070 or www.interactiveimagery.com.

Notes

1. C. and S. Simonton, and J. Creighton, *Getting Well Again* (Los Angeles: Tarcher, 1978).

2. E. Rossi, *The Psychobiology of Mind/Body Healing* (New York: W. W. Norton, 1986).

3. "Integration of Behavioral and Relaxation Approaches into the Treatment of Chronic Pain and Insomnia." NIH Technology Assessment Panel on Integration of Behavioral and Relaxation Approaches into the Treatment of Chronic Pain and Insomnia. *Journal of the American Medical Association* 276, no. 4 (July 24–29 1996): 313–318.

4. H. L. Bennet, D. R. Benson, and D. A. Kuiken. "Preoperative Instructions for Decreased Bleeding during Spine Surgery," *Anesthesiology* 65, (1986): A245.

5. D. Hathaway, "Effects of Preoperative Instruction on Postoperative Outcomes: A Meta-Analysis," *Nursing Research* 35, (1986): 269–275.

6. R. B. Gremillion and R. F. van Vollenhoven, "Rheumatoid Arthritis. Designing and Implementing a Treatment Plan," *Postgraduate Medicine* 103, no. 2 (February 1998): 103–106, 110, 116–8.

7. J. R. Horton, "Clinical Hypnosis in the Treatment of Rheumatoid Arthritis," *Psychologische Beitrage* 36, nos. 1–2 (1994): 205–212.

8. F. I. Fawzy et. al., "Malignant Melanoma. Effects of an Early Structured Psychiatric Intervention, Coping, and Affective State on Recurrence and Survival 6 Years Later," *Archives of General Psychiatry* 50, no. 9 (September 1993): 681–689.

9. D. Spiegel, "Mind Matters. Coping and Cancer Progression," *Journal of Psychosomatic Research* 50, no. 5 (May 2001): 287–90.

10. D. Spiegel et. al., "Group Psychotherapy for Recently Diagnosed Breast Cancer Patients: A Multicenter Feasibility Study," *Psychooncology* 8, no. 6 (Nov–Dec. 1999): 482–493.

11. R. P. Blankfield, ap., "Suggestion, Relaxation, and Hypnosis as Adjuncts in the Care of Surgery Patients: A Review of the Literature," *American Journal of Clinical Hypnosis* 33, no. 3 (January 1991): 172–186.

12. D. Bresler, *Free Yourself from Pain.* (New York: Simon & Schuster, 1979).

13. R. N. Jamison, W. C. Parris, and W. S. Maxson. "Psychological Factors Influencing Recovery from Outpatient Surgery," *Behaviour Research and Therapy* 25 (1987): 31–37.

14. D. R. Daake, "Imagery Instruction and the Control of Post-Surgical Pain," *Applied Nursing Research* 2, no. 3 (August 1989): 114–120.

CHAPTER FOURTEEN

The Role of Spirit
in Healing

Len Saputo, M.D.

Traditionally, spirit has been revered as a vital and sacred element of the healing process in indigenous and historical cultures world-wide. Spiritual teachers have passed their secrets of healing from generation to generation for thousands of years. The obvious reason for this is that spiritual practice can ease suffering and promote healing. Yet, relieving symptoms is only the first step in real healing.

Ancient healers believed that there is purpose for everything in the universe and that this is true of illness as well. By understanding this purpose, they found that it is possible to realize deeper meaning in the lives of individuals and even of entire communities. Disease is regarded as more than physical disability and psychological challenge; rather it is thought of as an opportunity to learn more about who we are and as a tool to move us forward on our spiritual path.

Today, we are "going back to the future." Many Americans are encouraging their health-care practitioners to include spiritual practice as part of their treatment. There are several reasons why this is occurring. Despite the remarkable achievements of modern technology, we live in an era that is plagued by an epidemic of chronic diseases. Almost 50 percent of Americans have at least one chronic disease, and things are getting worse.[1] We're at a point where we're willing to do whatever it takes to find solutions to this dilemma.

Humanity has relied on spirituality for healing for millennia and continues to have great faith in the value of this approach. Abundant research in medical journals documents that people who have strong faith, religious belief, or a spiritual practice enjoy better physical, mental, and emotional health. In our efforts to heal, we want to explore every aspect of who we are and any approach to healing that may help us become (or remain) healthy. The holistic nature of body, mind, and spirit are aspects of our fundamental nature, and each domain offers a window through which we can promote healing.

We Americans are reclaiming our responsibility to take care of our own health. We want to collaborate with our health-care professionals and also actively participate in our own healing by choosing the therapies we use. We have awakened to what our ancestors have always known — that healing is the return wholeness.

Returning to Spirituality

There is a growing appreciation by the medical profession that both spirituality and human connection are important aspects of health and healing. In ancient times, health care and spiritual guidance were believed to be so intimately interrelated that a single practitioner, the priest, midwife, or shaman, usually provided both of these aspects of healing. However, as medicine has become based more on science and less on what we have always intuitively known, physicians have focused on science and released spirituality to religion. Modern medicine is reawakening to the importance of both science and spirit and is looking for ways to merge these inseparable perspectives in healing.

Holistic medicine is once again emerging. A recent medical review of more than 1,200 studies supports this trend.[2] At least two-thirds of these studies document significant associations between religious activity and better mental health, better physical health, or lower use of health care services.

A survey of 1,000 American adults reported that 79 percent believed that spiritual faith could help people recover from disease.[3] Sixty-three percent felt it was the responsibility of physicians to address spiritual issues. In perhaps the most well-known studies on alternative medicine in the United States, Harvard Medical School's David Eisenberg, M.D., reported that 25 percent of interviewees stated they used prayer as an adjunct to standard medical therapy.[4,5] In a study of hospital inpatients, 48 percent stated that they would like their physician to pray with them.[6] *The Journal of Family Practice* found in a survey of 203 hospitalized patients that 94 percent believed spiritual health is as important as physical health and that 73 percent prayed daily.[7]

Today, there is a rapidly growing body of scientific literature documenting the value of this ancient wisdom. Research confirms that patients who actively participate in spiritual practice are much more likely to recover from a serious illness than those who do not.[8,9,10,11,12,13,14] Americans have always believed in spiritual or religious practice, and now that there is mounting scientific evidence supporting its value, we are relying on it even more to assist us in many areas of health care.

Almost thirty U.S. medical schools now include training in religion and spirituality.[15] Our physicians are increasingly recognizing the importance of prayer. In a survey of 296 physicians of the American Academy of Family Physicians, 99 percent stated they believed that religious beliefs could heal, and 75 percent believed that the prayers of others (intercessory prayer) could promote healing in a patient.[16]

We are a very fortunate generation. Never before in history have we had the opportunity to merge the miracles of modern technology with the miracles of spiritual healing traditions. The movement to include spirituality in medicine is being led by physicians such as Larry Dossey, Herbert Benson, Bernie Siegel, James Gordon, Rachel Naomi Remen, Martin Rossman, and many others. Where does spirit fit into building good health and strong immunity?

Connecting with Spirit

There are many definitions of spirituality. In this book, spirituality refers to the universal consciousness through which we are all connected. The soul is the spark of spirit instilled in each of us that is the essence of who we are and that connects us to universal consciousness.

The mind or intellect, on the other hand, is a human quality that is composed of both intellectual and emotional faculties. It is what fuels our creativity. The mind is not the primary focus in indigenous cultures; it is just one component of humanity. In today's culture we deify the mind, placing it on a pedestal. In the process, we may compromise the opportunity for spiritual balance. Coming into spiritual balance is not a mental process; it does not involve the mind. In fact, the mind is most often an obstacle in this process, since the experience of pure consciousness occurs in a state of silence, devoid of thought or language.

One of our biggest challenges as human beings is to move out of our minds and go inward, so that we can hear our spiritual voice. This is not easy, because the ego wants to stay in control. When we release the illusion of being in control, we surrender to a place of humility. When the mind quiets, we become more open to connecting with spirit. The openness to receive new possibilities germinates from the humility of being willing to exist in a place of "not knowing." There is a timeless place within that can put you in touch with the peace of a quiet mind and in connection with spirit. It is in this setting that we don't have to *do* anything — the wisdom passes into us from outside. We become a vessel that holds information, transferred to us. Lao-tzu once wrote:

> Empty yourself of everything. Let the mind become still. The ten thousand things rise and fall while the Self watches their return. They grow and flourish and then return to the source. Returning to the source is stillness, which is the way of nature.

There are many tools that can help us connect with spirit. The range is nearly as infinite as the diversity within humanity — we're all different, and we each make that connection in our own special way. Yet, our needs are much the same; we're looking for connection with others and with the universal life force. The approach you choose will depend on what appeals to you. You may also discover new approaches that you didn't imagine could be of interest.

In the tradition of the shaman, our purpose in life is to restore our wholeness in the context of all aspects of our entire existence. This healing process is revered as our sacred journey within. Examples of healing techniques that can quiet the mind and connect us with spirit include:

- Prayer
- Spiritual practice or worship
- Meditation
- Relationships and community
- Communion with nature
- Guided imagery
- Music and sound therapies
- Art
- Dance and movement therapies
- Meditative exercise (yoga, Qigong, and t'ai chi)
- Breathing exercises
- Chanting
- Sweat lodges and vision quests
- Connecting with spirit through laughter or touch

Prayer

Prayer is a powerful tool that can help you get your mind out of the way to connect with spirit. There are a multitude of studies documenting that religious participation, especially through prayer, is associated with improvement in many diseases. Studies have been done showing that among patients with a wide variety of chronic conditions, those who are the most spiritually connected have the best outcomes.[17]

One of the most fascinating and compelling studies on the effects of prayer was done at San Francisco General Hospital in 1988 by Dr. Randolph Byrd.[18] In this widely quoted study, Dr. Byrd studied 393 patients in the coronary care unit and divided them into two groups. Both groups received appropriate medical treatment. However, the second group also received intercessory prayer through prayer groups. When the outcomes of the two groups were compared, those prayed for had more favorable outcomes in five specific areas:

- Less incidence of congestive heart failure
- Fewer cases of cardiac arrest
- Less pneumonia
- Decreased need for antibiotics
- Less need for additional medical procedures

In another remarkable study, patients with advanced AIDS were prayed for and considered with positive intention. The focus of the study was "remote healing" (healing from a distance).[19] Although there were no significant changes in levels of immune cells, the prayed-for patients experienced beneficial clinical results that included:

- Reductions in new complications of AIDS
- Reductions in the severity of their disease
- Less need for visits from medical personnel
- Fewer hospitalizations

Intercessory prayer has also been documented to benefit patients with rheumatoid arthritis, showing improvements in symptoms and physical signs such as swollen and tender joints, and laboratory results.[20] Patients with long-standing and moderately severe arthritis were shown to have significant improvements from intercessory prayer. For the next twelve months, those patients experienced:

- Pain reduction
- Less fatigue
- Improved function of joints
- Reduced joint swelling

Spiritual Practice or Worship

Spiritual practice has been associated with improved health in general. A recent scientific study assessed spiritual well-being in patients with coronary heart disease and correlated this with progression or regression of their disease.[21] During a four-year period, it was determined that those patients with the lowest levels of spiritual well-being had the most progression of coronary artery disease. Spiritual practice was found to confer significant protection against the progression of disease.

Meditation

Medical research has documented that people who meditate regularly also enjoy better health, have stronger immune systems, are more aligned with their purpose in life, and are more relaxed. Dean Ornish, M.D., is probably most famous for his pioneering work in the treatment of disease through lifestyle interventions. His research has documented that it is possible to reverse coronary heart disease through a medically supervised program of meditation, regular exercise, and a vegetarian diet.[22] An interesting finding in these studies revealed that the single most powerful determinant predicting how well patients with heart disease would do was related to whether or not they felt interconnected. Patients who tended to use the words *we, our,* and *us* as opposed to those who used *I, me, my,* and *mine* were less likely to experience progression of their disease.

Whether or not people perceived themselves to be alone or interconnected had a significant effect on whether their heart disease progressed or regressed.

Relationships and Community

Relationships are a link to the divine, acknowledged in many religions. For example, Quakers honor "that of God in every man." It is not surprising that good relationships are a vital component of health and that they become extra important when we are ill. A number of major studies have confirmed this. In New York, researchers tracked the progress of more than seven hundred people with serious illness and found that coping and improvement paralleled the adequacy of social support from family, friends, and others in their lives, even after all significant variables were taken into account. Research at Stanford has found that women with breast cancer who participated in support groups lived twice as long as those without social support. The best of our relationships reflect the embodiment of our spirituality.[23]

Communion with Nature

We also have a sacred relationship with nature, and it can serve as a powerful healer. In our own ways, we are each an integral part of its collective wholeness. Nature, too, offers a sacred relationship with us. By accepting her invitation, our relationship deepens. Connecting with nature can be very restorative. This sense of reconnection can occur through any activity that places us in a natural environment — walking by a river, smelling the fresh forest rain, or even just watching clouds in the midst of a crowded city. These experiences bring us more in tune with spirit, reminding us that we are a part of all that is, and always have been.

Guided Imagery

Chapter thirteen is devoted to the powerful applications of imagery in connecting with spirit and in healing. For a more detailed review, you may also want to refer to Dr. Rossman's book, *Guided Imagery for Self-Healing.*

Music and Sound Therapies

Great music has the ability to bring us into harmony with spirit. The language of tones, rhythm, and form allows us to deeply and simultaneously communicate within ourselves and with one another. This resonance creates a sense of unity that can be not only awe inspiring but also truly healing. The messages of great composers can transcend the conscious mind and reach us at a soul level, bringing us into more perfect balance with universal spirit. Most of us have experienced this remarkable phenomenon. The music that nourishes our soul may vary from Bach to African drumming, from choral music to world music.

We have been musical beings since before recorded history. Rhythm and sound have always been used in the expression of our feelings, and these messages have extended across time, cultures, religion, and politics. Music is a universal language. How music affects us is not fully understood, but we all appreciate that its effects can be relaxing, energizing, depressing, joyous, annoying, or romantic and can induce most every known emotion. Music is also a powerful tool to help us clear the mind and enter a meditative state and has been used for millennia to help us connect with spirit.

Recent scientific research has documented that our physiology is influenced by music; the adrenal glands and immune system are significantly affected. For example, studies of ceremonial drumming have shown beneficial changes in stress hormone levels and heightened immune factors.[24] Studies of the effects of music on patients with cancer have shown that music can increase their sense of well-being and of relaxation. These studies also documented increased levels of antibodies and decreases in the stress hormone cortisol.[25]

As a doctor, Frances was one of the early victims of AIDS.
That was before the dangers of a simple needle stick were known. At the time, there was little to be done about it. The drugs helped, but not enough. But music! She got a Walkman, put together a first-rate collection of tapes, and began immersing herself in a world of music. It didn't heal her, but it did transform the quality of her life.

Art

Our own creative expression can put us in touch with intense psychological and creative energy and enable us to tap a deep vein of power that is difficult to describe. The artistic medium could be anything that is meaningful, anything we enjoy and do well at. Robert Shuman, an insightful psychologist who battles multiple sclerosis, suggests, "Art can bring the possibility of healing to those living with illness. One purpose of art is to give form to that which is unspeakable, to render coherent the shattered and broken. Just as illness can [negate] experience, art can give it both spirit and flesh. Art is a medicine for the suffering we call illness."[26]

Dance and Movement Therapies

Motion and rhythm are primary characteristics of all life forms; they begin very early in intrauterine life and continue to have a profound effect on our health and well-being throughout life. Movement marks the beginning and end of life. In fact, without movement there can be no life. How we move reflects not only our thoughts and feelings but also the expression of our spirit. This is a reflection of the inseparable nature of body, mind, and spirit.

At their deepest level, movement therapies are holistic spiritual practices that become a way of life. They are powerful tools that bring our attention to being in the moment, reminding us of our interconnectedness with the entire universe, our oneness.

Movement disciplines balance the two hemispheres of the brain, bringing together the linear and creative, the analytical and the emotional, and open us to connection with spirit. Movement, music, and ritual also remind us that indigenous and ancient cultures have used variations of these forms of expression to honor our inseparable connection to one another as well as to everything in the universe. Ancient healing disciplines celebrate the expression of body, mind, and spirit through movement. Through movement we reconnect to spirit.

Meditative Exercise

More than 80 million people practice therapeutic forms of exercise such as yoga, Qigong, and t'ai chi daily in India, China, and worldwide. These holistic practices have been documented to improve most chronic health conditions ranging from hypertension to diabetes. They combine balanced slow movement with deep breathing to increase physical vitality. They are perhaps best known for their ability to reduce stress and enhance immunity. (See chapter 5 for more information on meditative exercise.)

These practices offer some of the same benefits as classic meditation. Of yoga it has been said, "There is nothing to do, only to 'un-do,' in order to return to wholeness. Yoga is the remembrance of the unity and oneness that we already are."[27] There are several ways that connection to spirit manifests through yoga. This system is intended to be adapted to each individual and their needs. The physical practices of hatha yoga are expressed through various exercises described as asanas. Through this practice, we can increase our attunement to the eternal cosmic vibration by bringing our attention more fully into the present and through concentration on our breathing. Each yogic posture can become a physical expression of prayer. It also creates the release of habitually contracted muscles, which opens and expands our awareness to the oneness of the inner cosmos and outer cosmos.

Breathing Exercises

Breathing is much more than a simple mechanical act. Today there is a growing interest in the relationship of breathing to both health and spiritual development. All ancient indigenous healing systems consider the breath a source of life-force energy that brings healing energy into the body. The use of the breath is very integral to the practice of many disciplines, including yoga and Ayurveda, Taoism, Zen, and Tibetan Buddhism. Contemporary health-care practitioners are making an effort to revive these methods of breathing. These practices promote deeper relaxation and self-awareness, improved management of stress, and enhanced health and wholeness. When we are in this state of deep relaxation and the mind slows down, it is much easier to connect with spirit.

There is an intimate and inseparable relationship between our emotional state and how we breathe. It has been documented that the degree of acidity or alkalinity (pH) of our blood determines not only how our cells operate but also how we think and feel.[28] By working with a "breathing coach" it is possible to retrain our style of breathing to bring about more ideal physiology as well as a more relaxed mind and body.

Most bodyworkers appreciate that breath, emotion, and body posture are so interrelated that collectively they reflect who we are. Through the use of certain forms of massage coupled with breathing exercises, emotional and spiritual issues may come into the conscious awareness, offering the opportunity of dealing with them more fully. Important aspects of the physiology of breathing that relates to optimal health are beginning to be understood.

Chanting

Chanting is integral to most ancient forms of spiritual practice, ranging from Christian Gregorian chants to Tibetan practices. It is a form of prayer that facilitates quieting mental chatter, transcending the mind, opening the heart, and connecting with spirit. Sound, tone, and rhythm are often combined in a synergistic way with breath and movement to achieve connection with spirit. Chanting is a way to produce healing vibrational frequencies of sound. Over the millennia, it has been observed that each chakra system has a specific healing frequency of sound. This encourages a rebalancing and purification that brings us back to what we are and always will be — that is the oneness that we all are.

Sweat Lodges and Vision Quests

In the Native American tradition, ceremony is regarded as a very powerful way to receive help from the spiritual dimension. The vision quest is a sacred individual ceremony wherein the seeker journeys to a natural place and sits alone for one to four days in prayer and meditation, awaiting a vision to be revealed. These visions are used to guide personal development and to facilitate healing.

The sweat lodge is a purification ceremony designed to provide physical and spiritual cleansing. Sweating promotes the discharge of toxins from the body. Even more important, participants are guided to look inward and confront their deepest conflicts. The physical challenge imposed by the extreme heat encourages transcendence from the physical and mental to the spiritual domain. As inner conflicts surface, they can then be released. This tradition has served Native Americans for ten thousand years and is still available for those who would like to experience this mode of healing.[29]

Laughter

The healing effects of laughter and positive emotional states have been found to enhance immune function and encourage healing. It also brings us into the moment, connecting us with our inner self. Norman Cousins, in his book *Anatomy of an Illness,* described how he used laughter and nutritional therapy to heal from a severe joint disorder. Since Dr. Cousins's initial work, this approach has been successfully integrated into guided imagery, hypnotherapy, and other meditative states that have been shown to provide powerful healing benefits. Our state of mind has a strong influence on our body and its ability to heal.

Touch

Touch is a basic human need. Infants who don't receive touch may not survive or develop normally. We need human contact even more when we are ill. In addition to being soothing, touch can unlock painful memories stored in the muscles and tissues of our body, through treatment called somatic therapy. We've all heard of how the mind affects the body through "psychosomatic" illness. This can work in reverse as well: Treating the body can heal the mind. A variety of bodywork techniques can not only make us feel physically and mentally nourished but can also encourage healing on a deeper level. "Mind-body medicine" has become a popular approach during the past decade, and therapies such as the Alexander Technique, Feldenkrais, Rosen method bodywork, craniosacral therapy, and many others have been documented to heal the mind through manipulation of the body. The deep relaxation that is associated with these therapies quiets the mind and brings us into connection with spirit.

Healing as a Sacred Journey

Traditionally, the very process of healing is regarded as a sacred journey within. Illness may bring us back to our basic values, the importance of the people in our lives, and the spiritual aspects of life. When we are challenged by illness, we tend to become more oriented toward fundamentals. We are reminded of the significance of our relationships. We realize the limited nature of the material side.

In essence, illness can play an important role by awakening us to our spiritual purpose. Illness can be seen as an opportunity for spiritual transformation rather than physical disability and psychological challenge. This is not always easy. We may feel disinclined to engage in this dimension of our life. We may become totally consumed with fixing the illness and have little energy left to search for spiritual transformation. Most of us consider it asking a lot to make spiritual transformations even when we are well!

Nonetheless, chronic illness can become an opportunity for spiritual growth. When we're ill, our most immediate concern is to be "cured" of our illness. We want to operate with a perfect body and feel good again. We seek out health-care practitioners who promise to deliver these services and highly value their work. Clearly this is an intelligent approach. However, it is also possible to look at the meaning of illness in the context of who we are as unique individuals, determine what it represents in our whole life story, and prosper from the journey through it. This can place great demands on our patience, especially when we are suffering. Yet illness can be valued as a transformative opportunity that presents the possibility of evolving further on our spiritual path. Connection with spirit can make the deepest context of healing a reality.

Even though curing the body and healing the soul are not the same, they can occur simultaneously. They are not mutually exclusive. We deserve nothing less.

Deepening the Journey

1. Now that we have explored various ways of connecting with spirit, it is possible to begin putting this information to work and deepening your experience of this process. Choose one of the styles of connection that appeals to you, and prepare to begin your inner journey.

2. Connecting with spirit is natural, and we often do so without noticing that this is what we are doing. You know that inner voice that guides you to take a certain action or make an important decision. Go there. For most people, being in a quiet place where it is easy to relax and "let go" facilitates this. However, what works is often different for each of us. It could happen when we are immersed in the beauty of a wondrous vista, but it could also happen

during the intensity of a tennis match, or during meditation. It is about being fully focused in the "precious present." After all, that is all there is — the past is over, and the
future does not yet exist.

3. You are inseparably interconnected with the universe. You
   are part of it, and it is part of you. Experience what it feels
   like to be supported and to support at the same time. Let
   your imagination explore this feeling — let go and notice
   the oneness that emerges.

4. As we become engaged in the busyness of everyday life, it
   is easy to lose sight of our spiritual nature. Imagine how
   it might feel to be part of the universal community. When
   you are connected with spirit, you will sense your deepest
   connection to life.

5. In the final analysis, our connection with spirit is about
   love — love for ourselves, our friends, and all that there is.

᠍ᢒᢧ

Len Saputo, M.D., is founder and president of the Health-Medicine
Forum, a network of more than three thousand health-care professionals that provides information on complementary and alternative
medicine for both health-care professionals and a broad public
audience. Dr. Saputo is also medical director of the Health
Medicine Institute, Walnut Creek, California. Patient appointments
and consultations can be arranged by calling (925) 937-9550.

Notes

1. C. Hoffman, D. Rice, and Hai-Yen Sung, "Persons with Chronic
   Conditions: Their Prevalence and Costs," *Journal of the American Medical
   Association* 276 (1996): 1473–1479.

2. H. G. Koenig et al., *Handbook of Religion and Health: A Century of Research
   Reviewed* (New York: Oxford University Press, 2000).

3. T. McNichol, "The New Faith in Medicine," *USA Today,* April 7, 1996, p. 4.

4. D. M. Eisenberg, R. C. Kessler, C. Foster et al., "Unconventional Medicine in the United States," *New England Journal of Medicine* 328 (1993): 246–252.

5. D. M. Eisenberg, R. B. Davis, S. L. Ettner et al., "Trends in Alternative Medicine Use in the United States, 1990–1997, *Journal of the American Medical Association* 280 (1998): 1569–1575.

6. D. E. King and B. Bushwick. "Beliefs and Attitudes of Hospital Inpatients about Faith Healing and Prayer," *Journal of Family Practice* 39 (1994): 349–352.

7. B. B. King, D.E., "Beliefs and Attitudes of Hospital Inpatients about Faith Healing and Prayer," *Journal of Family Practice* 39, no. 4 (1994): 349–352.

8. D. Larsen, M. G. Milano, and C. Barry, "Religion: The Forgotten Factor in Health Care," Website www.worldandi.com/subscribers/1996/february/index.shtml, accessed February 1996.

9. G. W. Comstock and K. B. Partridge, "Church Attendance and Health," *Journal of Chronic Diseases* 25 (1972): 665–672.

10. T. E. Oxman, D. H. Freeman, and E. D. Manheimer, "Lack of Social Participation or Religious Strength and Comfort as Risk Factors for Death after Cardiac Surgery in the Elderly," *Psychosomatic Medicine* 57 (1995): 5–15.

11. L. Dossey, *Healing Words: The Power of Prayer and the Practice of Medicine* (San Francisco: HarperCollins, 1993).

12. L. Dossey, *Recovering the Soul: A Scientific and Spiritual Search* (New York: Bantam Books, 1989).

13. D. Ornish, *Love and Survival: The Scientific Basis for the Healing Power of Intimacy* (New York: HarperCollins, 1998).

14. D. B. Larson, *The Faith Factor, Volume Two: An Annotated Bibliography of Systematic Reviews and Clinical Research on Spiritual Subjects* (Bethesda, Md.: National Institute for Healthcare Research, 1993).

15. J. S. Levin, D. N. Larson, and C. M. Puchalski, "Religion and Spirituality in Medicine: Research and Education," *Journal of the American Medical Association* 278 (1997): 792–793.

16. F. B. Daaleman, T.P., "Spiritual and Religious Beliefs and Practices of Family Physicians: A National Survey," *Journal of Family Practice* 48 no. 2 (1999): 98–104.

17. J. Kass et al., "Health Outcomes and a New Index of Spiritual Experience," *Journal of Scientific Study and Religion* 30 (1991): 203–211.

18. R. B. Byrd, "Positive Therapeutic Effects of Intercessory Prayer in a Coronary Care Unit Population," *Southern Medical Journal* 81 (1988): 826.

19. F. Sicher, E. Targ, D. Moore et al., "A Randomized Double-Blind Study of the Effect of Distant Healing in a Population with Advanced AIDS: Report of a Small-Scale Study," *Western Medical Journal* 169 (1998): 356.

20. D. A. Matthews et al., "Intercessory Prayer Ministry Benefits Rheumatoid Arthritis Patients," *Journal of General Internal Medicine* 13, suppl. 1 (1998): 17.
21. E. M. Morris, "Relationship of Spirituality to Coronary Heart Disease," *Alternative Therapies* 5 (September/October 2001): 96–98.
22. D. Ornish et al., "Can Lifestyle Changes Reverse Coronary Atherosclerosis?" *Hospital Practice* 26, no. 5 (1991): 123–126, 129–132.
23. D. Spiegal et al., "Effect of Psychological Treatment on Survival of Patients with Metastatic Breast Cancer," *The Lancet* (October 14, 1989): 888–891.
24. B. Bittman et al., "Composite Effects of Group Drumming Music Therapy on Modulation of Neuroendocrine-immune Parameters in Normal Subjects," *Alternative Therapies* 7, no. 1 (January 2001): 38–47.
25. S. I. Burns et al., "A Pilot Study into the Therapeutic Effects of Music Therapy at a Cancer Help Center," *Alternative Therapies* 7, no. 1 (January 2001): 48–56.
26. R. Schulman, *The Psychology of Chronic Illness* (New York: Basic Books/HarperCollins, 1996).
27. R. Vernone, oral communication, Health Medicine Forum, Walnut Creek, Calif., 2001.
28. H. Aihara, *Acid and Alkaline* (Oroville, Calif.: George Ohsawa Macrobiotic Foundation, 1999).
29. L Mehl-Madrona, "Native American Medicine in the Treatment of Chronic Illness: Developing an Integrated Program and Evaluating its Effectiveness," *Alternative Therapies* 5, no. 1 (January 1999): 36–44.

CHAPTER FIFTEEN

Piecing the Puzzle Together

Len Saputo, M.D., and

Nancy Faass, M.S.W., M.P.H.

Lifestyle: Medicine of the Future

Wellness and prevention are the way of the future for primary health care. In prevention, the most important factors are related to how we live our lives — our lifestyle. Throughout the book, we've looked at research that documents the value of basic lifestyle factors such as sleep, exercise, water, food, stress, and connection to spirit. In some form, lifestyle has been an essential component of every major system of natural medicine throughout history and has been appreciated for thousands of years as the key to good health.

The purpose of this book is to provide you with the latest information on this approach. It translates into practical, safe, inexpensive tools you can apply in your own life. You can tailor these tools to meet your unique personal requirements. Lifestyle changes have the potential to:

- Stimulate stronger immunity
- Increase energy and vitality
- Enhance overall health

Medical research has made dramatic strides in identifying what we need to know to live longer and healthier lives. Much of the research deals with commonsense basics. The findings suggest practical strategies to achieve maximum wellness — using approaches that are available to everyone.

You can apply this information in your daily life with confidence, knowing that it is based on the latest findings and medical practice. We've taken great care to include viewpoints from health-care professionals of many disciplines. This integrative approach combines the best from both mainstream and complementary medicine.

We have also offered a holistic perspective, taking into account the whole person — body, mind, and spirit. This provides a broader range of approaches to healing. It also encourages a focus on the person rather than the disease process.

A Personalized Approach

The lifestyle factors reviewed in this book can be individualized to meet your specific needs. This is an opportunity to select approaches that feel right to you. Since we are all different, we encourage you to personalize the information that appeals to you. Adapt it to the unique requirements of your own physiology.

- How much sleep do you need?
- How much exercise?
- What is your ideal diet?
- Which resources are essential to maintain balance in your life?

When one has a chronic illness, factors as simple as diet and exercise may need to be modified with the health condition in mind, based on advice from your primary care provider. Even doctors don't treat themselves. We encourage you to find a health-care professional with whom you can develop a good working relationship. Sometimes it's important to get a second opinion.

Seek out a practitioner who is knowledgeable and highly informed and who will hear your deepest needs and concerns. It can be beneficial to see someone whose approach is holistic. You will want a seasoned health-care provider who has had experience with your particular type of problem. It is the interplay, the feedback between their wisdom and yours, from which the best strategies for your healing process are most likely to emerge.

Getting the Most from This Book

Consider applying these changes in lifestyle one at a time, and at your own pace. There is no hurry. Track your progress by keeping a record and noticing what happens. Chances are you will benefit even if you only do some of them. The changes you make for yourself are also likely to have a positive effect on those around you.

One way to apply this book is to periodically review each chapter and, one chapter at a time, gradually integrate the information into your life. To keep track of your progress, you may want to record and measure changes through a log, food diary, or a journal. You can monitor your success by asking:

- Do I feel better after making that change?
- Is there more vitality in my life?
- Has my endurance improved?
- Has my energy increased?

Maximum Health

We all want to get the most out of living. So there is tremendous value in increasing the awareness of how we live our lives. It is also important to take action. We can learn to use lifestyle as a tool. This could make the difference between enjoying health or struggling with illness. These approaches to lifestyle are straightforward and realistic. We also want to encourage you to explore other complementary therapies in your search for the best possible health. Consider supplementing the information in this book with other resources. Every change you incorporate into your daily life will help you enjoy better health and greater vitality.

We wish you well.

Resources

General Resources

How to Find More Information on Your Own

Listed here you will find both general resources on immune health as well as resources on specific topics covered in the chapters of this book.

Books

Bock, Kenneth, M.D., and Nellie Sabin. *The Road to Immunity: How to Survive and Thrive in a Toxic* World. New York: Pocket Books, 1997.

Clough, Nancy Coe, and James A. Roth. *Understanding Immunology.* St. Louis: Mosby, 1997.

Sompayrac, Lauren M. *How the Immune System Works.* Malden, Mass.: Blackwell Science, 1999.

Patient Information Resources
Medline Database

Summaries from the medical literature are available online at PubMed, a service of Medline, the database of the National Library of Medicine at the National Institutes of Health at www.nlm.nih.gov/pubmed.

Research Services

Institute for Health and Healing Library (formerly Planetree Health Resource Center), 2040 Webster Street, San Francisco, CA 94115; phone (415) 923-3681; email: ihhlib@sirius.com.

The Heath Resource, 933 Faulkner Street, Conway, AR 72032; phone (800) 949-0090; email: moreinfo@theheathresouce.com.

World Research Foundation, 41 Bell Rock Plaza, Sedona, AZ 86351; phone (520) 284-3300.

Referrals to Practitioners

American Academy of Environmental Medicine, 7701 E. Kellogg, Suite 625, Wichita, KS 67207; phone (316) 684-5500.

The American Association for Health Freedom, 459 Walker Road, Great Falls, VA 22066; phone (703) 759-0662; practitioner referrals available at www.atma.nic.

American Association of Naturopathic Physicians, 8201 Greensboro Drive, Suite 300, McLean, VA 22101; phone (703) 610-9037; fax (703) 610-9005; Website www.naturopathic.org.

American Association of Oriental Medicine, 433 Front St., Catasauqua, PA 18032; phone (610) 266-1433.

American Chiropractic Association, 1701 Clarendon Blvd., Arlington, VA 22209; phone (800) 986-4636; Website www.amerchiro.org.

American College for the Advancement of Medicine, P.O. Box 3427, Laguna Hills, CA 92654 (Send an envelope with two stamps.); phone (800) 532-3688.

American Holistic Medical Association, 6728 Old McLean Village Dr., McLean, VA 22107; phone (703) 556-9728; Website www.holisticmedicine.org.

American Holistic Veterinary Medical Association, 2218 Old Emmorton Rd., Bel Air, MD 21015; phone (410) 569-0795; Website www.ahvma.org; email office@ahvma.org.

Bastyr University Referral Line, Kenmore, WA; phone referrals to naturopathic physicians who have attended Bastyr available by calling (425) 602-3390.

Metagenics Gig Harbor, P.O. Box 1729, Gig Harbor, WA 98335; referrals to physicians and practitioners trained in functional medicine available by calling (800) 843-9660.

National Center for Homeopathy, 801 N. Fairfax Street, Suite 306, Alexandria, VA 22314; phone (703) 548-7790; Website www.homeopathic.org.

Orthomolecular Health-Medicine Society, 2698 Pacific, San Francisco, CA 94115; phone (415) 922-6462.

Additional Resources by Chapter

Chapter 3: Are You Getting Enough Sleep?

Books

Dement, William C., M.D., Ph.D., and Christopher Vaughan. *The Promise of Sleep*. New York: Dell, 1999. Includes a listing of every major clinic in the United States that provides treatment for sleep disorders.

Walsleben, Joyce A. et al. *A Woman's Guide to Sleep: Guaranteed Solutions for a Good Night's Rest*. New York: Times Books, 2000.

Wiley, T. S. with Bent Formby. *Lights Out*. New York: Pocket Books, 2000.

Websites

W B & A Market Research. 2001 Sleep in America Poll. Washington, DC: National Sleep Foundation, 2001; Website www.sleepfoundation.org.

Chapter 4: What about Water?

Books

A'o, Lono Kahuna Kupa. *Don't Drink the Water*. Pagosa Springs, Colo.: Kali Press, 1996.

Batmanghelidj, Fereydoon. *Your Body's Many Cries for Water*. Falls Church, Va.: Global Health Solutions, 1995.

Keegan, Lynn and Gerald T. Keegan, M.D. *Healing Waters*. New York: Berkley Books, 1998.

Ross, Julia. *The Diet Cure*. New York: Penguin, 2000.

Ryrie, Charlie. *The Healing Energies of Water*. Boston: Charles Tuttle Co., 2000.

Information on Municipal and Country Water

Call your county water department.

Call EPA's Safe Drinking Water Hotline: (800) 426-4791.

Contact the Environmental Defense Fund at www.scorecard.org.

Contact the Environmental Working Group at www.ewg.org

Information on Testing Tap or Well Water

Spectrum Laboratories, St. Paul, MN; phone (800) 447-5221. Call for information on lead and bacteria testing.

Suburban Water Testing, Temple, PA; phone (800) 433-6595. Call for information on testing for bacteria, fluoride, lead, nitrates, and other substances.

Information on Bottled Water and Water Filters
Clean Water Action; phone (202) 895-0420.

Consumer Reports, July 1997.

Environmental Working Group, Washington, DC; Website www.ewg.org.

International Bottled Water Association (IBEW), Virginia; phone (800) 928-3711. Provides information on quality of bottled water.

NSF International, Consumer Affairs Department, Ann Arbor, MI; phone (800) 673-6275; consumer guides to water filters and bottled water.

Request testing information directly from the vendor before you purchase monthly service.

Chapter 5: Getting Your Immune System in Shape
Qigong and T'ai Chi Books and Videos
Cohen, Ken. *The Way of Qigong.* New York: Ballantine Books, 1997.

Douglas, Bill. *The Complete Idiot's Guide to T'ai Chi and Qigong.* New York: MacMillan Publishing Company, 1999.

Garripoli, Francesco. *Qigong: the Essence of the Healing Dance.* Deerfield Beach, Fla.: Health Communications, 1999.

Huang, Chungliang Al. *Embrace Tiger, Return to Mountain.* Berkeley, Calif.: Celestial Arts, 1987.

Immune Enhancement Project of San Francisco. *Qigong for Health,* video. For phone orders, call (415) 863-9213.

Jahnke, Roger. *The Healing Promise of Qi.* New York: Contemporary Books, 2002.

———. *The Healer Within.* San Francisco: HarperCollins, 1999.

———. *Awakening the Medicine Within,* video. Health Action, 1995. For phone orders, call (800) 824-4325.

Liang, Shou-Yu. *Qigong Empowerment.* East Providence, R.I.: Way of the Dragon, 1996.

Lowenthal, Wolfe. *There Are No Secrets.* Berkeley, Calif.: North Atlantic Books, 1991.

Qigong Websites
HealthWorld Online: www.qigong-chikung.com.

Jahnke, Roger: www.healerwithin.com.

National Qigong Association: www.nqa.org.

Qi Journal: www.qi-journal.com.

Yoga Books, Journals, Videos, and Audiotapes
Birch, Beryl Bender. *Power Yoga: the Total Strength and Flexibility Workout.* New York: Fireside, 1995.

Christensen, Alice. *The American Yoga Association Beginner's Manual.* New York: Fireside, 1997.

Honig, Meenakshi. *Yoga Feels Good,* video. Wellbeing International. (800) 367-9642.

Iyengar, B. *Yoga: The Path to Holistic Health.* New York: Dorling-Kindersley, 2001.

Kabat-Zinn, Jon. *Full Catastrophe Living: Using the Wisdom of Your Body and Mind to Face Stress, Pain, and Illness.* New York: Delta-Dell Books, 1990.

Ornish, Dean, M.D. *Dr. Dean Ornish's Program for Reversing Heart Disease.* New York: Ballantine Books, 1990.

Schiffmann, Eric. *Yoga: The Spirit and Practice of Moving Into Stillness.* New York: Pocket, 1996.

Stress Reduction Tapes. *Mindfulness Meditation,* audiotape. The University of Massachusetts, under the guidance of Jon Kabat-Zinn, offers a set of audiotapes with hatha yoga exercises (Series One tapes). The tapes can be ordered from Stress Reduction Tapes, P.O. Box 547, Lexington, MA 02420 or by checking their Website www.minfulnesstapes.com.

Yoga Journal. Phone (510) 841-9200; Website www.yogajournal.com.

Walking Books and Magazines

Fenton, Mark. *The 90-Day Fitness Program.* New York: Perigee, 1995.

Iknoian, Therese. *Fitness Walking.* Champaign, Ill.: Human Kinetics, 1995.

Jordan, Peg. *The Fitness Instinct.* Emmaus, Pa.: Rodale Press, 2000.

Malkin, Mort. *Aerobic Walking, the Weight-Loss Exercise.* New York: Wiley, 1995.

Prevention Magazine. Phone (800) 763-2531.

Chapter 6: Purification
Books and Videos

Ballentine, Rudolph, M.D. *Radical Healing.* New York: Harmony Books, 1999.

Barnard, Neal, M.D. *Foods that Fight Pain.* New York: Three Rivers Press, 1998.

Cutler, Ellen, M.D. *The Food Allergy Cure.* New York: Harmony Books, 2001.

————. *Winning the War against Asthma and Allergies.* Albany, N.Y.: Delmar Publishers, 1998.

————. *Winning the War against Immune Disorders and Allergies.* Albany, N.Y.: Delmar Publishers, 1998.

————. *Creating Wellness,* video. Larkspur, Calif.: BioSET, 2001.

D'Adamo, Peter J. *Live Right for Your Type.* New York: Putnam, 2001.

————. *Eat Right for Your Type.* New York: Putnam, 1996.

Krohn, Jacqueline, M.D., and Frances Taylor. *The Whole Way to Natural Detoxification.* Vancouver, B.C.: Hartley and Marks, 1996.

Kushi, Aveline. *Aveline Kushi's Complete Guide to Macrobiotic Cooking.* New York: Warner Books, 1989.

McCarty, Meredith. *American Macrobiotic Cuisine*. New York: Penguin/Putnam, 1996.

Milne, Robert, M.D., and Blanke More, with Burton Goldberg. *An Alternative Medicine Definitive Guide to Headaches*. Tiburon, Calif.: Future Medicine Publishing, 1996.

Murray, Michael T. *Chronic Fatigue Syndrome*. Rocklin, Calif.: Prima Publishing, 1994.

Resources

BioSET, Institute P.O. Box 5356, Larkspur, CA 94977; phone (877) 927-0741; fax (415) 945-0465; Website www.bioset-institute.com; email biosetseminars@aol.com. Information on BioSET products, practitioners, newsletters, and seminars for the public and professionals.

Environmental Purification Systems, P.O. Box 191, Concord, CA 94522; phone (510) 284-2129. Water filtration products.

Greenpeace Guide at www.truefoodnow.org/shopping list. This Website lists thousands of everyday food products and indicates whether they contain genetically altered ingredients.

Infrared saunas. Phone (877) 839-0125; Website www.massageclinic.com.

Metagenics Customer Service, San Clemente, CA; phone (800) 692-9400; Website www.metagenics.com. UltraClear nutritional supplements are available from health-care practitioners and can be ordered from Metagenics.

WellZyme. Phone (800) 228-1501; Website www.wellzymes.com.WellZyme enzymes are beneficial for detoxification.

Chapter 7: Digestion — The Best-Kept Secret
Books and Newsletters

Berkson, D. Lindsey, and Jonathan Wright. *Healthy Digestion the Natural Way*. New York: Wiley, 2000.

Bland, Jeffrey, and Sara Benum. *The 20-Day Rejuvenation Diet Program*. New York: McGraw Hill-NTC, 1996.

Galland, Leo. *Power Healing*. 2d. ed., New York: Random House, 1998.

Gates, Donna, and Linda Schatz. *The Body Ecology Diet: Recovering Your Health and Rebuilding Your Immunity*. Atlanta, Ga.: B.E.D. Publications, 1997.

Gittleman, Ann Louise. *Guess What Came to Dinner*. New York: Penguin/Putnam, 1994.

Health On-Line at www.healthonline.com. See the monthly online newsletter by Dr. Leo Galland, which often discusses issues on digestive health.

Lipski, Elizabeth. *Digestive Wellness*. New York: McGraw Hill-NTC, 2000.

Nichols, Trent, M.D., and Nancy Faass. *Optimal Digestion.* New York: HarperCollins, 1999.

Schmidt, Michael A., Lendon H. Smith, and Keith W. Sehnert. *Beyond Antibiotics.* Berkeley, Calif.: North Atlantic Books, 1994.

Trenev, Natasha. *Probiotics: Nature's Internal Healers.* New York: Penguin/Putnam. 1998.

Testing Information for the Public and Health-Care Professionals

BioHealth Diagnostics. San Diego, CA. Lab test panels and consultation; phone (800) 570-2000.

Great Plains Laboratory, Overland Park, KS. Organic acids testing; phone (913) 341-8949.

Great Smokies Diagnostic Lab, Ashville, NC. Testing for functional status of hormones, liver, and digestive health; phone (800) 522-4762; website www.gsdl.com.

Immuno Laboratories, Fort Lauderdale, FL. Food allergy testing; phone (800) 231-9197.

SpectraCell Laboratories, Inc., Houston, TX. Testing for levels of vitamins, minerals, fatty acids; phone (800) 227-5227.

Chapter 8: Eating Your Way to Health
Books

Bland, Jeffrey. *Genetic Nutritioneering.* New York: McGraw Hill-NTC, 1999.

Crook, William, M.D.. *The Yeast Connection Handbook.* Berkeley, Calif.: Professional Books, 1999.

Daoust, Gene and Joyce. *The Formula.* New York: Ballantine, 2001.

———. *40-30-30: Fat Burning Nutrition.* Del Mar, Calif.: Wharton Publishing, 1996.

Wolever, Thomas S. et al. *The Glucose Revolution: The Authoritative Guide to the Glycemic Index.* New York: Marlowe and Company, 1999.

Sears, Barry. *The Zone.* New York: Regan Books, 1995.

Steward H., M.D., et al. *Sugar Busters.* New York: Ballantine, 1998.

Werbach, Melvyn R., M.D. *Nutritional Influences on Illness,* 2d. ed. Tarzana, Calif.: Third Line Press, 1993.

Consultations

Lifespan Institute, 524 San Anselmo Avenue, #106, San Anselmo, CA 94960. Nutritional and anti-aging programs; testing and telephone consultations; phone (415) 479-3552.

Chapter 10: Clearing Toxins

See Resources under chapter six.

Chapter 11: Minimizing Your Exposure to Toxins

Books and Magazines

Anderson, Jeffry, M.D., and Jerry Stine. "Detoxing from Toxins." In Nichols, Trent, MD, and Nancy Faass. *Optimal Digestion.* New York: HarperCollins, 1999.

Ashford, N. A. and C. S Miller. *Chemical Exposures: Low Levels and High Stakes.* New York: Van Nostrand Reinhold, 1997.

Berthold-Bond, Annie. *Clean and Green.* Woodstock, N.Y.: Ceres Press, 1994.

———. *The Green Kitchen Handbook.* New York: HarperCollins, 1997.

Colborn, Theo, Dianne Dumanoski, and John Myers. *Our Stolen Future.* New York: Dutton, 1996.

Dadd, Debra. *Home Safe Home.* New York: Tarcher/Putnam, 1997.

Haas, Elson. *The Staying Healthy Shopper's Guide.* Berkeley, Calif.: Celestial Arts Press, 1999.

Moses, Marion. *Designer Poisons.* San Francisco: Pesticide Education Center, 1995.

Organic Gardening, Rodale Press, Emmaus, Pa. (800) 763-2531.

Rogers, Sherry A., M.D. *Chemical Sensitivity.* New York: McGraw-Hill, 1995.

———. *Tired or Toxic?* Syracuse, N.Y.: Prestige Publishers, 1990.

Steingraber, Sandra. *Living Downstream.* Reading, Mass.: Addison Wesley, 1997.

———. *Having Faith: An Ecologist's Journey to Motherhood.* New York: Perseus Books, 2001.

Steinham, David. *The Safe Shopper's Bible: A Consumer's Guide to Nontoxic Household Products, Cosmetics, and Food.* New York: MacMillan, 1995.

Winter, Ruth. *A Consumer's Dictionary of Food Additives.* New York: Three Rivers Press, 1999.

Organizations and Referrals to Practitioners

The American Academy of Environmental Medicine, 7701 E. Kellogg, Suite 625, Wichita, KS 67207; phone (316) 684-5500. Conferences, workshops, and training; books, abstracts, monographs, and audiotapes; referrals to physicians of environmental medicine.

The American Environmental Health Foundation, Dallas, TX; phone (214) 361-9515; (800) 428-2343. Extensive resource center and mail-order catalog for educational books, abstracts, and audiotapes; treatment strategies; environmentally safe products for the home and personal care.

The Chemical Injury Information Network, White Sulphur Springs, MT; phone

(406) 547-2255; Website www.biz-comm.com/CIIN. Education, research, and advocacy related to chemical injury; extensive referral resources, monthly newsletter, research services, and educational materials.

The Cutting Edge, Southampton, NY; phone (800) 497-9516. Product catalog.

Environmental Dental Association (EDA). P.O. Box 2184, Rancho Santa Fe, CA 92067; phone (800) 388-8124. For book orders, call (619) 586-7626. To receive a list of alternative dentists, send three dollars in a self-addressed stamped envelope with fifty-five cents' postage.

Advocacy Organizations for the Environment

The Bio-Integral Resource Center (BIRC), P.O. Box 7414, Berkeley, CA 94707; phone (510) 524-2567.

E Magazine, Subscriptions, Marion, OH; phone (800) 967-6572.

Environmental Working Group, Oakland, CA; phone (510) 444-0973; Washington, DC; phone (202) 667-6982; Website www.ewg.org.

Mothers and Others: Website www.mothers.org.

National Resources Defense Council, Washington, DC; phone (202) 289-6868; San Francisco, CA: phone (415) 777-0220; New York: phone (212) 727-2700; Los Angeles, CA: phone (323) 934-6900; Website www.nrdc.org.

Pesticide Action Network of North America (PANNA), San Francisco, CA; Website www.panna.org/panna/.

Chapter 12: Dealing with Stress
Books and Journals

Baker, Sidney M., M.D. *The Circadian Prescription*. New York: Putnam Publishing Group, 2001.

Bland, Jeffrey, Ph.D. *Disorders of Intercellular Mediators and Messengers: Their Relationship to Functional Illness*. Gig Harbor, Wash.: Institute for Functional Medicine, Inc., 1999.

———. *Improving Intercellular Communication in Managing Chronic Illness*. Gig Harbor, Wash.: Institute for Functional Medicine, Inc., 1999.

Galland, Leo, M.D. *Power Healing*. New York: Random House, 1998.

Jeffries, William M., M.D. *Safe Uses of Cortisol*. Springfield, Ill.: Charles C. Thomas Publishers Ltd., 1996.

Kabat-Zinn, Jon. *Full Catastrophe Living: Using the Wisdom of Your Body and Mind to Face Stress, Pain, and Illness*. New York: Delta, 1990.

Khalsa, Dharma Singh, M.D., and Cameron Stauth. *The Pain Cure*. New York: Warner Books, 1999.

Selye, Hans, M.D. *The Stress of Life*. New York: McGraw-Hill, 1956.

Tunn S., et. al., "Simultaneous Measurement of Cortisol in Serum and Saliva after Different Forms of Cortisol Administration." *Clinical Chemistry* 38, no. 8 (1992): 1491–1494.

Vining RF, and others. "The Measurement of Hormones in Saliva." *Journal of Steroid Biochemistry.* 27 (1987): 81–94.

Websites

Diagnostechs, Inc., Kent, WA; Website www.diagnostechs.com; information on saliva testing for cortisol.

Great Smokies Diagnostic Laborabories, Asheville, NC; Website at www.gsdl.com; information on saliva testing for cortisol.

Consultations

Lifespan Institute, 524 San Anselmo Avenue, #106, San Anselmo, CA 94960. Nutritional programs that address stress and hormone issues. Testing and telephone consultations; phone (415) 479-3552.

Chapter 13: Imagine Health

Books

Rossman, Martin, M.D. *Guided Imagery for Self-Healing.* Tiburon, Calif.: H. J. Kramer/New World Library, 2000.

———. *Healing Yourself: A Step-by-Step Program for Better Health through Imagery,* 2d ed. Mill Valley, Calif.: The Academy for Guided Imagery, 1997.

Consultations

Martin Rossman, M.D., Mill Valley, CA; phone (415) 383-3197. Available for phone consultations on health conditions and also the use of mind-body approaches to resolve them.

Resources and Training for the Public and Professionals

The Academy for Guided Imagery, Mill Valley, CA; phone (800) 726-2070. A free catalog of relaxation tapes, imagery tapes, and videos. Referrals to practitioners available through the *Directory of Imagery Practitioners;* information on classes and groups where you can refine your skills at www.interactiveimagery.com.

The Institute of Transpersonal Psychology, Palo Alto, CA; phone (650) 493-4430; Website www.itp.edu. Offers training in the many uses of imagery, including its applications in healing.

Chapter 14: The Role of Spirit in Healing
Books

Bolen, Jean Shinoda. *Close to the Bone.* New York: Simon & Schuster; 1998.

Cousins, Norman. *Anatomy of an Illness.* New York: Bantam, 1995.

Dalai Lama. *The Art of Happiness.* New York: Riverhead, 1998.

Myss, Carolyn. *Why People Don't Heal and How They Can.* New York: Random House, 1998.

Ornish, Dean, M.D. *Love and Survival: Eight Pathways to Intimacy and Health.* New York: HarperCollins, 1998.

Remen, Rachel Naomi. *Kitchen-Table Wisdom.* New York: Berkeley Trade, 1997.

Rossman, Martin L., M.D. *Guided Imagery for Self-Healing.* Tiburon, Calif.: H J Kramer/New World Library, 2000.

Ruskan, John. *Emotional Clearing: A Groundbreaking East-West Guide to Releasing Negative Feelings and Awakening Unconditional Happiness.* New York: Broadway Books, 2000.

Shuman, Robert. *The Psychology of Chronic Illness.* New York: Basic Books/HarperCollins, 1996.

Resources

Fields Book Store, 1419 Polk Street, San Francisco, CA 94109; phone (415) 673-2027; books on the world's great spiritual traditions, including the connection of mind and spirit to healing on the Web at www.fieldsbooks.com.

Index